KT-222-537

Normalisation

Normalisation, the theoretical framework that underpins the movement of services for people with disabilities from long stay hospitals, has recently become the focus of much academic and professional attention. As the community care debate has moved into the public arena, it has attracted a certain amount of criticism, and is beginning to acknowledge the political and philosophical conflicts that surround it.

Normalisation: A Reader for the Nineties provides a much needed, informed appraisal of this controversial philosophy and combines various perspectives on the subject, including applied behavioural analysis, social policy and psychodynamic approaches. Thus it explores the discrepancies between the ideal and the reality and extends the debate by drawing comparisons with other political and social ideologies.

This book will be invaluable to professionals working with people who have mental health problems, learning difficulties or physical disabilities. It will be of interest to health care workers, students of social work, social policy and administration, psychology and occupational therapy.

Hilary Brown is Senior Lecturer in Mental Handicap and **Helen Smith** is Lecturer in Mental Health at the Centre for Applied Psychology of Social Care at the University of Kent. They are both widely experienced and have published on the subject of normalisation and its surrounding issues.

Normalisation
A reader for the nineties

Edited by
Hilary Brown and Helen Smith

Foreword by Linda Ward

MORNINGSIDE SITE LIBRARY
LOTHIAN COLLEGE OF HEALTH STUDIES
CANAAN LANE
EDINBURGH
EH10 4TB.
Tel: 0131 536 5616/5617

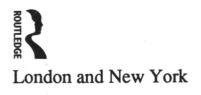

London and New York

LIBRARY	LOTHIAN COLLEGE OF HEALTH STUDIES
CLASS	WM 872
ACC No.	174758
DATE	29 11 95
PRICE	£12-99

CA 362.380941 BRO.

First published 1992
by Routledge
11 New Fetter Lane, London EC4P 4EE

Simultaneously published in the USA and Canada
by Routledge
29 West 35th Street, New York, NY 10001

Reprinted 1993

© 1992 Hilary Brown and Helen Smith

Typeset in Times by LaserScript, Mitcham, Surrey
Printed and bound in Great Britain by
Mackays of Chatham PLC, Chatham, Kent

A Tavistock/Routledge Publication

All rights reserved. No part of this book may be reprinted or
reproduced or utilized in any form or by any electronic,
mechanical, or other means, now known or hereafter
invented, including photocopying and recording, or in any
information storage or retrieval system, without permission in
writing from the publishers.

British Library Cataloguing in Publication Data
Normalisation: a reader for the nineties.
  1. Mentally disordered persons. Rehabilitation
  I. Brown, Hilary *1949–* II. Smith, Helen *1958–*
  362.2

Library of Congress Cataloging in Publication Data
Normalisation: a reader for the nineties/edited by Hilary Brown and
  Helen Smith; foreword by Linda Ward.
  p. cm.
  1. Mentally handicapped – Care – Great Britain. 2. Community mental
  health services – Great Britain. I. Brown, Hilary, 1949– .
  II. Smith, Helen, 1958– .
  HV3008.G7N67 1991
  362.3′8′0941 – dc20   91-12881
                                                                       CIP

ISBN 0–415–07079–1
ISBN 0–415–06119–9 (pbk)

Contents

Contributors

Hilary Brown has worked in residential services for people with learning difficulties in this country and in the United States and more recently as a trainer in Health, Social Services and the Voluntary Sector. She has a special interest in issues around sexuality and people with learning difficulties and is the author of several training packages, including the Lifestyles Materials and Bringing People Back Home video-assisted packs. She is currently Senior Lecturer in Mental Handicap at the Centre for the Applied Psychology of Social Care, University of Kent.

Gillian Dalley is a research fellow at the Policy Studies Institute. She has previously worked in the Centre for Health Economics, York and the King's Fund. Her interests include community care and the assessment of quality in health and social care. She is currently working on social security issues.

Eric Emerson trained and worked as a clinical psychologist in this country and in Canada, specialising in learning difficulties. Before joining the Hester Adrian Research Centre, University of Manchester, as Senior Research Fellow, he worked at the University of Kent and South East Thames Regional Health Authority. His interests are in behaviour analysis, challenging behaviours, normalisation and the evaluation of services for people with learning difficulties. He is currently working on a study examining behavioural processes underlying challenging behaviours and on two projects, evaluating the quality and costs of locally based support teams for people with challenging behaviours and a residential educational service for adults with multiple sensory impairments and severe learning difficulties.

Peter Ferns is currently an independent trainer and consultant and was until recently a Training and Development Manager at the London

Boroughs Training Consortium (LBTC). He has worked in residential and day-care services for people with learning difficulties for many years. He has a particular interest in race equality and social work education and has been involved in several initiatives to develop a Black perspective and anti-racist practice in social work.

Peter Lindley is a Service Development Consultant and a Research Associate based at the Centre for the Applied Psychology of Social Care, University of Kent. He has worked in mental health services all his career. He has extensive experience of teaching, research and management. His particular interests include services for people with long-term mental health problems, consumer participation and training in dispersed community services.

Peter McGill has a joint appointment with the University of Kent and South East Thames Regional Health Authority as Senior Lecturer in Social Psychology of Mental Handicap and Special Development Team Leader. He has several years' experience in services for people with learning difficulties, having worked in health, social services and the voluntary sector in a variety of roles – as instructor, residential social worker and clinical psychologist. His current work focuses on services development and staff training around people with severe learning difficulties and challenging behaviour.

Helen Smith has a joint appointment as a lecturer in mental health in the Centre for the Applied Psychology of Social Care at the University of Kent and training adviser in mental health services for South East Thames Regional Health Authority. Previously she worked in mental health services development for the King's Fund Centre. Her professional background is as a clinical psychologist in adult mental health services. Her current interests are in service design and quality assurance, particularly with services for people with long-term mental health problems.

Sue Szivos worked in Social Work with people with learning difficulties before completing a first degree in Philosophy/Psychology at Exeter University. She then completed a Ph.D. on the self-concept of people with learning difficulties in which she examined the social comparisons made by people with learning difficulties and their feelings about their handicap and stigmatisation. These issues remain of interest to her. Her other interests include ideology and its dissemination, communication and staff training. She currently holds a post as lecturer/training adviser in mental handicap at the University of Kent at Canterbury.

Alan Tyne taught in schools for ten years before joining 'Campaign for the Mentally Handicapped' (now VIA - 'Values into Action') as research and information officer. In 1979 with Paul Williams and Morag Plank he founded the sister-organisation CMHERA to develop a programme of normalisation-based training and service-evaluation in the United Kingdom. Since 1988 he has developed an independent programme of work called 'Constructive Options'. Through this he works alongside handicapped people, their families and friends, co-operating with services and community organisations to seek better futures in ordinary communities.

Tony Wainwright is the district clinical psychologist for Cornwall Health Authority. He was previously involved in the reprovision of services which had traditionally relied on a Victorian mental hospital which is scheduled for closure in 1992. After graduating in zoology, he gained his doctorate in experimental psychology in 1973. He has worked with people with long-term mental ill health since gaining his clinical qualification in 1981.

Simon Whitehead is currently Deputy Director of the National Developments Team for People with a Mental Handicap. He qualified as a social worker following a first degree in Sociology and a masters degree in social policy. After working as a social worker in Westminster, Berkshire and Derbyshire, he became involved in policy formulation and service developments, both in Derbyshire, and more latterly Suffolk, where he became First Assistant Director of Social Services.

Foreword

Linda Ward

It is more than ten years now since the birth of the 'Ordinary Life' movement in the UK. Taking its name from the first of a series of influential publications emanating from the King's Fund Centre in London, the message of the movement has been simple. People with severe learning difficulties can (and should) live their lives in the community like anyone else. The means of achieving this? Simple too: ordinary houses in ordinary streets (King's Fund Centre 1980); ordinary jobs in ordinary workplaces (King's Fund Centre 1984; Porterfield and Gathercole 1985); ordinary friends, neighbours, social and leisure opportunities (King's Fund Centre 1988) with whatever support is needed to enable this to happen.

Ten years on it is hard to conceive the enormous scepticism which greeted these ideas. People with severe learning difficulties, living in *ordinary* houses? Now that scepticism is largely gone. Experience has shown the impossible to be possible after all (even if it can be difficult). Throughout the UK such developments have become, if not common, then at least commonplace.

The principles of normalisation have been a driving force behind the Ordinary Life movement. Service planners, managers and staff have redrafted regional, district and local service plans, not to mention operational policies of individual houses, to embody normalisation principles and practices based upon them. People have tried to change not only their theory, but their practice. There has been much welcome change. But . . .

Inevitably, with a philosophy or set of principles as powerful as those involved here, there will be buts . . . . Normalisation has been a compelling force for positive change in services for people with learning difficulties in this country. But, as people have wrestled with trying to implement the principles of normalisation on the ground, some causes for concern have emerged. Mostly, the disquiet and the challenges have been muted. There has been a tacit understanding that if you're *for* normalisation and its positive influences on changing services for devalued people, then you should not argue *against* it publicly in any way. To do so, is to throw your weight behind the forces of reaction – or at least the forces which continue to work against the proper integration of disabled people within our society. There has been a real risk that the baby would be thrown out with the bath water. That people wishing to open up the debate on normalisation, but feeling frustrated in their attempts to do so, would reject the philosophy itself.

Hence, the significance of this book. The principles of normalisation and their history are described here with great clarity. The positives of normalisation are recognised and its achievements applauded. But the problematic issues are not ducked. For those who have been committed to the principles of normalisation, but who have wrestled (often painfully and in private) with the dilemmas posed, it will be a source of great relief. The conservative thrust of some elements of normalisation; its potential as yet another source of abuse of power over devalued people; its apparent inability to encompass the different circumstances, aspirations and values of women, black people, disabled people and carers; its uncomfortable emphasis on change of the devalued individual rather than the society in which they live; its apparent denigration of relationships amongst disabled and devalued people – all are addressed in their complexity; alongside some positive suggestions for taking a revitalised normalisation forward in the 1990s. Normalisation carries with it a tradition of inaccessible language, but this is a stimulating, informative and, above all, readable book.

The next decade will not offer any easy solutions in the development of better services for devalued people. Alongside the technical complexities of implementing the NHS and Community Care Act, the realities of general economic constraints are beginning to mean the re-emergence of institutionalisation in some places, the abandonment of an Ordinary Life, if not in principle, then sadly, sometimes, in practice. This reader in normalisation will be a source of strength and ideas for all those involved in the struggle to ensure our society (and its services) are better able to meet the needs of those currently devalued by it in the testing times that lie ahead.

REFERENCES

King's Fund Centre (1980) *An Ordinary Life. Comprehensive Locally-based Residential Services for Mentally Handicapped People*, London: King's Fund Centre.
King's Fund Centre (1984) *An Ordinary Working Life. Vocational Services for People with Mental Handicap*, London: King's Fund Centre.
King's Fund Centre (1988) *Ties & Connections. An Ordinary Community Life for People with Learning Difficulties*, London: King's Fund Centre.
Porterfield, J. and Gathercole, C. (1985) *The Employment of People with a Mental Handicap. Progress towards an Ordinary Working Life*, London: King's Fund Centre.

Preface

ON THEORY

The purpose of theory is to clarify the world in which we live, how it works, why things happen as they do. The purpose of theory is understanding. Understanding is energizing. It energizes to action. When theory becomes an impediment to action, it is time to discard the theory and return naked, that is without theory, to the world of reality. People become slaves to theory because people are used to meeting expectations they have not originated – to doing what they are told, to having everything mapped out, to having reality pre-packaged. People can have anti-authoritarian intention and yet function in a way totally consonant with the demands of authority. The deepest struggle is to root out of us and the institutions in which we participate the requirement that we slavishly conform. But an adherence to ideology, to any ideology, can give us the grand illusion of freedom when in fact we are being manipulated and used by those whom the theory serves. The struggle for freedom has to be a struggle towards integrity defined in every possible sphere of reality, sexual integrity, economic integrity, psychological integrity, integrity of expression, integrity of faith and loyalty and heart. Anything that shortcuts us away from viewing integrity as an essential goal or anything that diverts our attention from integrity as a revolutionary value serves only to reinforce the authoritarian values of the world in which we live.

Extract from Dworkin, A. (1979) 'Look, Dick, look. See Jane blow it', published in *Letters from a War Zone* (1988) Martin Secker & Warburg Limited.

Acknowledgements

We would like to thank the contributors for their promptness and thorough-ness in preparing their chapters and Carol Whitwill for her work on the manuscript; we have particularly appreciated her attention to detail in the final stages of editing. Linda Ward of the Norah Fry Research Centre at the University of Bristol has been supportive throughout the project and we should like to thank her for agreeing to write the Foreword to the book. Ann Craft, of the University of Nottingham, was also generous with her support when we got stuck! Heather Gibson at Routledge has also given us consis-tent encouragement. We should also like to thank colleagues at the Centre for the Applied Psychology of Social Care for their interest and debate.

Hilary would like to thank Martin and Joe for their affection and support at home and Helen would like to thank Paul for his sense of humour and support at home.

Introduction

Hilary Brown and Helen Smith

This is a not a book about practice, a manual on how to implement better services for people with disabilities, nor even an account of the successes and failures of those who have been working towards that aim over the last twenty years. It is, instead, an unapologetic return to the theory which has underpinned our attempts to bring about, and maintain, change in human services. We do not see academic debate as an irrelevance or normalisation as a hot-house plant which needs to be shielded from scrutiny, sharing with Oliver the view that

> . . . [the] marginalisation of disabled people within society has been made harder precisely because of the marginalisation of disability within sociology, social anthropology and a variety of other academic disciplines.
>
> (Oliver 1990: xi)

Good theory, then, is essential to good practice, because, as we quote in the Foreword, 'The purpose of theory is understanding. Understanding is energizing. It energizes to action' (Dworkin 1979).

When Wolfensberger codified his observations about the conditions to which people with disabilities were subject in the institutions which were supposed to care for them, he made a quantum leap in the way service workers could understand the lives of people with disabilities in terms of their being a 'devalued' group. The clarity of his analysis did indeed provide energy for change and a vision of how things could be. Nonetheless, we believe the time is ripe for a reassessment of the theory. We now have considerable and varied experience of working with the ideas to bring to a critical re-evaluation of the principle and a whole new set of political and social realities to contend with in the struggle to win and maintain decent services on behalf of people with disabilities. Many people remain in institutional settings while others are isolated (alongside their carers) and ill-served in community facilities.

Moreover, we have been witnessing a period of unprecedented social change and realignment, and one which has seen the emergence of a number of movements whose agenda challenges the propensity for certain groups to be marginalised and devalued. Their experience and analysis can also shed light on the issues which people with disabilities face in seeking integration and respect.

As we enter the 1990s, both health and social services' provision for people with disabilities, that is, for people in mental distress, with learning difficulties (mental handicap), physical disability or the problems associated with ageing, are undergoing great change. These changes are both political and social in nature and are occurring within a context that reflects the growing interest in community-based alternatives to institutionalised settings. The political agenda has been characterised by the move towards an internal market within health and local authority services, a split in the purchasing and providing of care and a marked growth in the use of a mixed economy, that is, public and private sector services.

These developments are paralleled by changes in social policy and clinical practice in regard to the delivery of care. Over the past thirty years, the large psychiatric and mental handicap hospitals have been reducing the number of long-stay beds and many are now in the final throes of closure. Community care has developed as a more humane and effective alternative for people with long-term and/or severe disabilities and is increasingly accepted by the general public. An ICM poll for the *Guardian* (23 July 1990) found that 69 per cent of those interviewed thought that the quality of life for people with mental illness would be 'a lot better in the community' and 55 per cent thought that wherever possible 'they should live in the community and be treated as out-patients when necessary'. For people with learning difficulties, there is overwhelming acceptance of their right to live in their own neighbourhood and indeed, services for this particular group have long been offered on a community basis. Services for elderly people, previously based mostly in Old Peoples Homes, are being replaced by domiciliary services wherever feasible and the number of long-stay psychogeriatric beds in institutions is diminishing as hospitals close. It is only services for people with physical disabilities that remain comparatively under-developed in both hospital and community settings.

There were many different motivations behind the shift away from institutional forms of care. The more cynically minded saw it as a cost-cutting exercise until subsequent revaluation of community care indicated that it was far from the cheap option initially assumed and, in some instances, proved more expensive. Old buildings were beginning to crumble and maintenance costs soar at the same time as land prices rose, turning institutional sites into prime development opportunities. Unionised labour and traditional working practices were challenged. Nevertheless, despite the incompatibility of the many stakeholders, a consensus has been forged and, whatever the separate agendas, community care is now largely considered to be the most appropriate form of care for people with disabilities.

Despite the widespread development of new services, there have been few relevant theoretical models from which to develop good practice. In fact, what has often happened is that institutional services have been physically relocated in the community, but little else about the nature of the service has changed. This has often been due to ignorance – professionals and other workers have generally not received adequate training to throw off the long historical legacy of institutionalised working practice and simply have not known how to offer different, more appropriate forms of care. Being in close contact with service users challenges staff to develop skills in teaching and in interacting in helpful ways, structuring daily activities so that people with disabilities can take back control over their lives. But this has not been as easy as the early optimism promised and has tested people's competence and commitment to the full.

Normalisation therefore offered a significant way of conceptualising the pull towards negative practice and an important model of how to reverse this. It is not an attractive word and has been much maligned and misunderstood! Early practitioners were confused as to whether it was people or settings which were to be made more 'normal' and the movement has been hindered by many unfounded assumptions. The prevalence of simplistic notions that normalisation meant 'to make people normal' led Wolfensberger to rename it 'social role valorisation', in an attempt to re-emphasise the centrality of supporting individuals in attaining socially valued roles rather than a spurious conformity. But the term has not caught on in this country, as Booth (1988) comments:

> I don't think I could be persuaded to use the term 'social role valorisation.' It is too far removed from my own ordinary language and hence appears to embody the professional mystifications which reduce the power of others to control their own lives.
>
> (Booth 1988: 107)

We have therefore used the term normalisation throughout the book to reflect its continued usage in this country.

Whether one is deciding on terminology or challenging aspects of the theory, writing about normalisation is no ordinary business. It has been developed and 'arbitrated' by a small group of very committed individuals and a strong peer group culture has grown up around it, including some and excluding others. Its use raises, for those wishing to write in this area, a whole series of seemingly trivial questions. Should it be spelt with a capital or lower case 'n', should it be spelt with a 'z' (American) or an 's' (British)? Is it a theory, a movement or a principle? Should we be using the term at all since Wolfensberger suggested the alternative 'social role valorisation?' These are not trivial issues, however, for the people involved with the normalisation network. The commitment and fervour which it can engender in individuals has led to it being likened to an evangelical movement, with associated doctrinal squabbles and schisms. This strength of feeling indicates that it is more of an ideology than a service technique.

As with any significant body of knowledge or ideas, choices have to be made about how they will be promulgated but also controlled, and normalisation is no exception. The wide range of misapplication led to a concern with 'purity' which resulted in close ties and supervision being maintained between the Training Institute in Syracuse where Wolfensberger had originally developed his version of normalisation (it is instructive to remember that he was himself branded a misunderstander on account of his significant departure from the tenor of the original Scandinavian model of the principle: see Perrin and Nirje 1985) and the movement which developed in this country to spread the ideas. This has had contradictory effects – on the one hand it has led to useful experience being shared internationally but on the other hand, it has blocked the development of a distinctive British movement and the integration of new perspectives into the model and the training. Despite widespread usage of the ideas in this country, surprisingly little has been written about normalisation and the literature which does exist focuses largely on implementation and practice, rather than on an analysis of the ideas through comparison with other models of change or political/social ideologies. Underpinning the development of normalisation is a powerful belief that this idea, or body of ideas, is owned by someone and therefore anyone who wishes to comment on it, to elaborate, contradict or embellish it, or raise new or different viewpoints, runs the risk of being seen to have 'got it wrong'. Thus, although Wolfensberger's work followed that of Nirje and Mikkelson, he has taken on an adjudicating role, correcting other people's misunderstandings and criticising their premises or presentation (see Wolfensberger 1980).

In drawing attention to this we do not wish to detract from the debt that is owed him for the quality and depth of his work and observations, but to question at what point an idea becomes common property to be redefined or reworked. What responsibility or right does the originator of a piece of work hold over the way it is subsequently used, abused or put into practice? The answers would seem to lie in the extent to which any work is ever the solitary product of an individual, as opposed to a synthesis of current debate and perspectives. We hope that the chapters in this book succeed in unravelling significant strands which run through the normalisation ideology but which are also rooted in other academic disciplines and movements for change. We have commented elsewhere that although normalisation is concerned with values, it is uncritical of its own roots in white, male, middle-class North American culture (Brown and Smith 1989). We feel the time has come to open up the debate rather than dampen it down.

Thus we believe that the dissemination of normalisation ideology has been flawed in that it has not taken full account of the diverse needs, experiences and modes of communication of those people, users, workers and carers who have a stake in services. The dominant ideology has focused on the reform of human services, but within this, gender, class and ethnicity have been obscured. These issues need to be addressed in terms of both the content of the theory and the process of training, the format of which has inadvertently alienated or kept away some women workers and stifled a debate which could have led to a strong sense of solidarity between them and the people they are working with. Meanwhile, men also may have suffered in being sent back, newly sensitised but unsupported, to their places of work, without exploring the issue of their own, usually privileged places in the hierarchies which perpetuate the conditions they had witnessed. The silence on these issues in the dissemination of normalisation, as in other studies of organisational change is

> an interesting example of ideology and how theoretical disciplines which attempt to uncover the underlying structures and systems of organisations can in doing so ignore the 'obvious'. This can be a convenient means to removing the obvious from contention, from political argument.
>
> (Hearn and Parkin 1987)

Recent developments suggest that some of these issues are being creatively tackled. John O'Brien's (1987) formulation of the five service accomplishments provides an agenda which does not make its own assumptions, or encourage those who share lives with people with disabilities to make assumptions, about how to enhance their lives. It enables service users, parents, family members and lay people to talk on equal terms with workers and service providers without jargon getting in the way. This is an important development as the complex language that underpins normalisation can form a barrier between those 'in the know', that is, those who have been on a PASS course, and those who have not. This language dynamic can be as effective in maintaining power over users, their families and direct care staff as the old institutional structures that normalisation seeks to overthrow.

This is not to say that the more complex ideas of normalisation are redundant. In managing service systems and monitoring the effects of political changes, such as those advocated in the free market service system, we must incorporate all that has been learned about the tendencies to warehouse and segregate people, the pulls away from thinking through a coherent model of what is being offered, the planning which is needed to ensure comprehensiveness of services available and the central commitment to evaluate services in terms of the kinds of networks, roles, contacts and activities which they make available to service users.

Normalisation will only meet these challenges, however, if it is fed by debate and encouraged to grow, expand and change to tackle the pertinent issues of the day. We are not talking about a debate in ivory towers, but one which involves all whose lives and work are affected by normalisation, including a rigorous academic analysis of the ideas in both the social policy and professional training fields, something which has been lacking until now. The words we use in such a debate and the manner in which it is conducted will determine whether or not it provides a useful stimulus to the enhancement of the lives of people with disabilities. Words carry meanings beyond those listed in the dictionary: consider, for example the impact of the term 'congregate' as opposed to 'communal' settings, and the material differences which are veiled by such euphemisms as 'informal' when what is meant is unpaid. Robinson (1989) complains of what he calls 'morally loaded rhetoric' and asks for 'an acceptance of open debate in which people can question aspects of normalisation without being treated as unprincipled fools or moral lepers' (Robinson 1989: 248). To disagree with aspects, or the whole of normalisation does not automatically mean a disavowal of community care (although some will in reality have that as their motivation); it can mean a desire to improve further the lives of people disempowered through their disability. Contributors to the book were chosen in the light of this continued commitment.

The book compares and contrasts normalisation with many different perspectives and ideologies. It focuses on services for people with learning difficulties and those for people with mental health problems; the generic term 'people with disabilities' is used throughout the book to refer to both user groups. The ideas are also relevant to services for elderly people and for people with physical disabilities; however, as normalisation has as yet made little impact on service delivery in these fields, they are not specifically included here for discussion.

Eric Emerson starts with a concise definition of the principle of normalisation and provides a historical account of the development of thought leading to our current understanding of the normalisation principle. His account of normalisation forms the basis of the following chapters.

Peter Lindley and Tony Wainwright explain how the teaching of normalisation has largely been through PASS workshops and critically examine how PASS works and its effects on individuals. The workshops are usually intense experiences for people and have been both praised and criticised for this reason. This chapter will address whether this is the most effective way of 'spreading the word'.

Alan Tyne powerfully reminds us that normalisation is only relevant if it improves and enhances peoples' lives. His account of the lives of some people who use services provides the backdrop to the ensuing discussion about the ideas. He traces its development as a social movement in this country and in so doing, extends the debate beyond the narrow boundaries of disability services.

Simon Whitehead undertakes a critical analysis of normalisation, highlighting the academic and political traditions on which it is based and the context within which it has gained credence.

The second section of the book looks at the compatibility of normalisation with other service models and with other ideologies.

First, Peter McGill and Eric Emerson explore the links and conflicts between normalisation and behavioural approaches. Normalisation presents a vision of what services *ought* to be achieving for people, and behaviourism has emerged as an important technique for how this vision might be reached – especially in services for people with learning difficulties. It is essential, therefore, to envisage how these two approaches might complement each other to bring about change.

Helen Smith and Hilary Brown (the editors) then go on to look at the links between an approach to change based on normalisation and an approach based on a psychodynamic understanding of the world. Each explores the way unconscious processes affect the way care is given and the interactions which take place between service users and workers. Psychodynamic concepts also explain institutional (mal)practices in terms of the protection they offered staff in the face of painful feelings and conflicts. These two approaches can be complementary when thinking about why people with disabilities are so devalued and when wanting to plan *successful* services based on the principle of normalisation.

Gillian Dalley contrasts the essentially individualistic approach to care inherent in normalisation-based services with a collectivist approach that has characterised other cultures in different places and times. She proposes the notion that modern social welfare policies have been motivated by competing ideologies – possessive individualism and collectivism – and places normalisation as implicitly supporting the current status quo of individualism.

Sue Szivos further defines the relationship between normalisation and individualism and explores the implications for individuals with disabilities, of community integration in normalisation terms. This chapter focuses on the role of collective action for service users, especially in regard to consciousness raising.

Peter Ferns describes how the assumption of homogeneity contained within the normalisation principle obscures the cultural diversity of people who use services. He clarifies the difference between racism and discrimination on the basis of disability and highlights the dangers of equating the two issues. He goes on to outline an interpretation of normalisation which is appropriate for our multi-racial society and which addresses the 'double discrimination' to which black service users are subject.

Hilary Brown and Helen Smith continue a critique of the values and norms underpinning normalisation through a feminist analysis of the ideas. They use feminist theory to draw out the similarities and the differences between the oppression and discrimination of women and that faced by people with disabilities, especially women with disabilities and their carers, paid and unpaid, the majority of whom are, of course, women.

The aim of the book is to break through the 'franchise model' of normalisation which exists currently and to stimulate debate about the principle and its implications for services. Normalisation is a sensitive and relevant approach to community care, but it raises conflicts and contradictions as well as commitment in seeking change. We wanted a debate which could be specifically British and address the particular issues which face disability services in the context of the demise of post-war welfarism. The work done by John O'Brien and the 'An Ordinary Life' work originating at the King's Fund Centre (the 'An Ordinary Life' series, 1982 onwards) was the start of such a process: the contributions in this book have been chosen in the hope that they will carry the principle into the 1990s, enabling us to protect services for vulnerable people in the new climate and develop innovative ways of empowering people with disabilities, as individuals and as a group.

A NOTE ON TERMINOLOGY

In this book we have taken the unorthodox step of referring to people who use community care services as 'people with disabilities'. Within this phrase we encompass specifically people with learning disabilities and people who use mental health services. Many of the ideas will also be relevant to people with physical disabilities and elderly people who are also sometimes in need of services and at risk of being stigmatised.

Our use of this generic term is designed to make the book more readable and *not* to confuse or downplay the distinct issues which are faced by these separate groups. We hope none of the groups referred to throughout the text will feel offended or oppressed by being referred to within this 'umbrella' phrase.

REFERENCES

Booth, A. (1988) 'Challenging conceptions of integration', in L. Barton (ed.) *The Politics of Special Educational Needs*, Lewes: Falmer Press.

Brown, H., and Smith, H. (1989) 'Whose Ordinary Life is it anyway? – a feminist critique of the normalisation principle', *Disability, Handicap and Society*, 4, 2: 105–19.

Dworkin, A. (1979) 'Look, Dick, look. See Jane blow it', in *Letters from a War Zone* (1988), London: Martin Secker and Warburg.

Hearn, J., and Parkin, W. (1987) *'Sex' at 'Work' – the power and paradox of organisation sexuality*, Brighton: Wheatsheaf.

King's Fund Centre (1980) *An Ordinary Life: Comprehensive locally-based residential services for mentally handicapped people*, London: King's Fund Centre.

King's Fund Centre (1984) *An Ordinary Working Life: Vocational services for people with mental handicap*, London: King's Fund Centre.

O'Brien, J. (1987. 'A guide to life style planning: Using the activities catalogue to integrate services and natural support systems', in B.W. Wilcox and G.T. Bellamy (eds) *The Activities Catalogue: An alternative curriculum for youth and adults with severe disabilities*, Baltimore: Brookes.

Oliver, M. (1990) *The Politics of Disablement*, London: Macmillan.

Perrin, B., and Nirje, B. (1985) 'Setting the record straight: A critique of some frequent misconceptions of the normalization principle', *Australian and New Zealand Journal of Developmental Disabilities* 11: 69–74.

Robinson, T. (1989) 'Normalisation: The whole answer?', in A. Brechin and J. Walmsley (eds) *Making Connections – reflecting on the lives and experiences of people with learning difficulties*, Milton Keynes: Open Uni- versity Press.

Wolfensberger, W. (1980) 'The definition of normalization – update, problems, disagreements, and misunderstandings', in R. Flynn and K. Nitsch (eds) *Normalization, Social Integration and Community Services*, Austin, Texas: Pro-ed.

1   What is normalisation?

Eric Emerson

The term normalisation has now been in use for three decades. During this period it has proven to be an influential concept in debates concerning the most appropriate way of providing services for people with learning difficulties in Scandinavia (for example, Bank-Mikkelsen 1980; Grunewald 1986), North America (for example, McCarver and Cavalier 1983; Pelletier and Richler 1982), the United Kingdom (for example, Tyne 1987, 1989) and Australasia (for example, Anninson and Young 1980). More recently, this influence has broadened to include other disability groups. Since the origination of the concept, in Denmark in the late 1950s, however, normalisation has been defined in a number of distinct ways. Indeed, there is really no such thing as *the* concept or principle of normalisation. Instead there exists a family of ideas that share a common ancestry but which diverge at critical points. In order to assess the impact or adequacy of the concept, therefore, it is necessary to disentangle this interlinked web in order to clarify which or whose notion of normalisation we are actually addressing. Indeed, one of the most abiding characteristics of the debate concerning the value or utility of the principle of normalisation has been the saddening extent to which criticisms have often been based upon gross mis-understandings regarding the actual meaning of the concept (cf. Wolfens-berger 1980a).

This chapter will attempt to identify the main formulations of normal-isation influential within the United Kingdom and to identify, for each of these strands, the characteristics and major implications for service provision.

THE DEVELOPMENT OF NORMALISATION: SCANDINAVIAN THINKERS – BANK-MIKKELSEN AND NIRJE

The concept of normalisation originated in Denmark where, in the 1959 Mental Retardation Act, the aim of services was defined as being 'to create an existence for the mentally retarded as close to normal living conditions as possible' (Bank-Mikkelsen 1980: 56).

This definition was later elaborated to include 'making normal, mentally retarded people's housing, education, working, and leisure conditions. It means bringing them the legal and human rights of all other citizens' (Bank-Mikkelsen 1980: 56). Throughout the 1960s this notion of normalisation came to have a considerable impact upon the development of services and associated enabling legislation for people with learning difficulties in both Denmark (Bank-Mikkelsen 1980) and Sweden (Nirje 1969) where normalisation was redefined as meaning

> making available to all mentally retarded people patterns of life and conditions of everyday living which are as close as possible to the regular circumstances and ways of life of society.
>
> (Nirje 1980: 33)

These early Scandinavian formulations of normalisation are reasonably straightforward in that they advocate that services should seek to maximise the quality of life of service users by reproducing the lifestyle experienced by non-disabled citizens. Nirje (1980) describes the key characteristics of such a lifestyle in relation to eight areas:

- *The rhythm of the day* including the times and patterns of waking, dressing, eating and retiring at the end of the day.
- *The rhythm of the week* which is described as including not only the demarcation of weekends as being different from weekdays but also the importance of enjoying home, work and leisure activities in different settings.
- *The rhythm of the year* including participating in vacations.
- *Progression through the stages of the life cycle* including exposure to the normal expectations of childhood, adolescence, adulthood and old age.
- *Self-determination.*
- *The development of heterosexual relationships* including the right to marry.
- *Economic standards* including equal access to benefit payments and fair wages for work undertaken in workshop settings.
- *Environmental standards* including the need for 'standards for physical facilities like schools, work settings, group homes and boarding houses ... [to] ... be modelled on those available in society for ordinary citizens' (Nirje 1980: 44).

While these two early definitions of normalisation may differ in some minor aspects (see Wolfensberger 1980a) their similarities are more important. In particular both approaches share three characteristics:

(1) they are egalitarian statements about the rights of service users;
(2) they focus on equality in terms of an individual's quality of life; and
(3) they do not specifically confront the issue of segregation in service design.

In these early definitions, normalisation becomes a statement about how services can reflect the basic rights of people with learning difficulties in an egalitarian society. As Perrin and Nirje point out 'normalization as originally defined is based upon a humanistic, egalitarian value base, emphasising freedom of choice and the right to self-determination' (Perrin and Nirje 1985: 71). Similarly, Bank-Mikkelsen suggests that 'a significant element of normalization theory is . . . the juridical and administrative view that all are equal under the law' (Bank-Mikkelsen 1980: 57). The grounding of normalisation in basic human and civil rights was reflected in the incorporation of the Scandinavian definition in the United Nations 1971 'Declaration of General and Specific Rights of the Mentally Retarded'. Thus, normalisation did not develop as an isolated ideal but reflected the prevalent liberal trends of many Western societies at that time to respond to the demand for the equal rights of a number of disadvantaged or minority groups.

The key point, however, is that normalisation for Nirje and Bank-Mikkelsen is about rights and, as such, requires no scientific justification. In addition to a basic emphasis on rightfulness, Bank-Mikkelsen and Nirje define normalisation in terms of the quality of life or lifestyle of service users. Bank-Mikkelsen (1980), for example, defines normalisation in relation to ensuring equality on a number of traditional social indicators of quality of life including housing, education, work and leisure. Nirje (1980), on the other hand, in taking a more psychological approach, defines the key aims of normalisation in terms of normative lifestyles.

The fundamental aim of normalisation in these early definitions was to ensure that people with learning difficulties enjoyed their rights to the same quality of life as non-disabled members of society. An implication of defining equality in these terms was that such equality *could* be pursued in settings which segregate service users from non-disabled citizens. Equality, at least in the short term, did not necessarily require integration. Bank-Mikkelsen, for example, argued that 'while normalization is the objective, integration and segregation are simply working methods' (Bank-Mikkelsen 1980: 56). Similarly, Nirje (1980) discussed the benefits of integrating people with severe learning difficulties with groups of people with mild or moderate learning difficulties.

As we shall see later, other commentators have tended to view the social integration of disadvantaged people as an essential component of normalisation based upon the belief, as Wolfensberger asserts, that 'in the long run, no good can come from any program ... that is not based on intimate, positive one-to-one relationships between ordinary (unpaid) citizens and those who are handicapped' (Wolfensberger 1980a: 77). However, the 'equal but separate' approach encapsulated in the Scandinavian definition was reflected in the initial impact of normalisation in the United Kingdom which occurred largely in relation to the design of the physical environment of essentially segregated services (for example, Centre on Environment for the Handicapped 1972; Gunzberg 1970; Gunzberg and Gunzberg 1973).

THE NORTH AMERICAN VERSION – WOLFENSBERGER

During the period in which the concept of normalisation was being developed in Scandinavia, significant changes were also beginning to occur in North America. The number of people in state and county psychiatric hospitals declined steadily from the mid-1950s onwards (Brown 1985). Civil rights activism at this time had resulted in the acknowledgement in Federal Courts of psychiatric patients' substantive right to treatment within the 'least restrictive alternative' (Castellani 1987). In 1963, John F. Kennedy called upon Congress for action

> to bestow the full benefits of our society on those who suffer from mental disabilities ... [and] ... to retain in and return to the community the mentally ill and mentally retarded, and there to restore and revitalize their lives.
>
> (cited in Scheerenberger 1983: 248)

A decade later Wolfensberger first proposed (Wolfensberger 1972) and then developed (Wolfensberger 1980a, 1980b; Wolfensberger and Glenn 1973a, 1973b, 1975a, 1975b; Wolfensberger and Thomas 1983; Wolfensberger and Tullman 1982) a more elaborate definition of normalisation in an attempt to 'North Americanize, sociologize, and universalize the Scandinavian formulations' (Wolfensberger 1980a: 7). He initially defined normalisation as the

> utilization of means which are as culturally normative as possible, in order to establish and/or maintain personal behaviors and characteristics which are as culturally normative as possible.
>
> (Wolfensberger 1972: 28)

This definition has undergone two main changes, reflecting first a growing emphasis upon the importance of the way in which disadvantaged people are portrayed or perceived by the public (Wolfensberger 1980a) and second, a reformulation of the aims of normalisation in terms of socially valued roles rather than culturally normative practices (Wolfensberger and Thomas 1983; Wolfensberger and Tullman 1982). Shortly after the introduction of the concept of valued social roles, Wolfensberger proposed renaming normalisation 'social role valorization' (Wolfensberger 1983a, 1984), a term which he defined as incorporating 'the most explicit and highest goal of normalization . . . .the creation, support, and defence of valued social roles for people who are at risk of devaluation' (Wolfensberger 1983a: 234).

Wolfensberger and Thomas (1983) identified seven core themes which were the theoretical underpinnings of normalisation.

1 The role of (un)consciousness in human services

Throughout Wolfensberger's writings (for example, Wolfensberger 1972, 1975, 1980a, 1980b, 1983a, 1987; Wolfensberger and Thomas 1983) there exists a powerful notion of social *intent* in historical and social processes. For Wolfensberger, social policies towards disadvantaged groups reflect 'society's real but destructive intentions or needs . . . [but that such] . . . unpleasant realities are apt to be denied and repressed into unconsciousness' (Wolfensberger and Thomas 1983: 25), not only by individuals but also by organisations and society as a whole. This view of society as some kind of cognate being is reflected in Wolfensberger's recent argument that society has

> made an identity alliance with death and . . . [is] working feverishly toward the destruction of life on this planet . . . [as reflected] . . . in a very well hidden policy of genocidal destruction of certain of its rejected and unwanted classes. . . . Once a society has made a decision (explicated or not) to come down hard on a devalued minority group, it will transact this decision through whatever technical measures it may take toward this group, even those measures that are interpreted as being to the latter's benefit.
>
> (Wolfensberger 1987: 141)

As a consequence of such an analysis, Wolfensberger places considerable emphasis upon raising the consciousness of those involved in human services by making manifest these latent social intentions.

2 The relevance of role expectancy and role circularity to deviancy-making and deviancy-unmaking

In his attempt to 'sociologize' normalisation, Wolfensberger (1972) combined the egalitarian aims of Bank-Mikkelsen and Nirje with some contemporary developments in sociology. During the 1960s and early 1970s,
societal reaction or labelling theories were playing a dominant role in the
sociological study of deviance. These theories proposed that the characteristics and behaviour of members of deviant social groups (for example,
people with disabilities or people who offend against the law) is largely
determined by the way in which society responds to them once they have
been 'labelled' rather than by any biological or psychological factors that
may have led the individual to become labelled in the first place. In other
words, once someone has been cast into a deviant social role 'the original
causes of the deviation recede and give way to the central importance of the
disapproving, degradational, and labelling reactions of society' (Lemert
1967: 17). As a result 'deviance is an *outcome* of societal reaction, or
labelling by official control bodies' (Davies 1975: 172, emphasis added).
As Scull points out, the notion that crime was largely caused by the criminal
justice system or that mental illness was largely the result of mental health
services were inherently attractive ideas in the radical 1960s and represented a refreshing challenge to the 'traditional notion that the societal
response to deviance represented no more than a benign and defensive
response to the presence of individual pathology' (Scull 1984a: 277).

These ideas provided the basic foundation for Wolfensberger's reformulation of normalisation. In particular, the notion that being cast into a
specific social role inexorably results in the individual fulfilling the expectations associated with the role is a dominant theme within normalisation
and social role valorization. Indeed, Wolfensberger states that

> it is a well established fact that a person's behavior tends to be pro-
> foundly affected by the role expectations that are placed upon him . . . .
> this permits those who define social roles to make self-fulfilling
> prophecies.
>
> (Wolfensberger 1972: 15–16)

Wolfensberger (1972) identified eight general roles that may be applied
to members of disadvantaged groups: subhuman organism, menace, un-
speakable object of dread, object of pity, holy innocent, diseased organism,
object of ridicule, eternal child. Consistent with societal reaction theory,
Wolfensberger and Thomas argue that the social expectations associated
with these roles constitute one of the

most powerful social influence and control methods known . . . [and, consequently] . . . these role expectancies have had predictably negative results, ie. devalued people by and large live up (or down) to these role expectancies, acting like animals or menaces.

(Wolfensberger and Thomas 1983: 25)

Wolfensberger does, however, show a concern for the limitations of such an analysis and warns that

overzealous proponents [of normalisation] are commonly guilty of the assumption that handicapped people are not handicapped, that retarded people are not retarded, and that every handicapped person could do and be almost anything if only provided with sufficient role expectancy and opportunity.

(Wolfensberger 1980a: 97)

Nevertheless, programmes for social action based on normalisation and social role valorization require services to place a central emphasis upon preventing service users being cast in damaging social roles and supporting or establishing them in positive or culturally valued social roles in all areas of life.

3 The 'conservatism corollary'

The 'conservatism corollary' suggests that a multiplicative relationship exists between the number of devaluing characteristics an individual may possess (or similarly, the number of devalued people in a group or setting) and their 'social visibility'. In other words the more devalued you are, the greater the impact of any further devaluing characteristic. Thus, for example, while many of us experience no approbation for minor eccentricities, for example, grown men playing with toy trains, people who are devalued would have their social identities significantly damaged if they were to engage in similar pursuits. As a result, normalisation suggests that services should *overcompensate* in order to minimise devaluing characteristics and establish social identities for users which are highly culturally valued rather than tolerated or simply ordinary.

4 The developmental model and the importance of personal competency enhancement

Inherent in normalisation since its inception in Scandinavia has been a commitment to view *all* individuals as being capable of growth and development. Within Wolfensberger's theorising, this focus upon enhancing the personal competence of service users is given additional emphasis due to the perceived importance of compensating for or reducing devaluing characteristics. Indeed, the basic aim of his formulation of normalisation is to establish people in valued social roles which, of course, are likely to demand skilled social or technical performance in a number of areas.

5 The power of imitation

Consistent with the general social-psychological flavour of societal reaction theory is the importance attached to imitation or modelling as methods of learning. According to Wolfensberger and Thomas 'imitation is one of the most powerful learning mechanisms known' (Wolfensberger and Thomas 1983: 26).

6 The dynamics of social imagery

At a more general level, Wolfensberger and Thomas argue that the generation and transmission of stereotypes about the characteristics of devalued or deviant groups take place largely through a process of the 'unconscious' association of social symbols or images. Thus, for example, it would be argued that the association in popular media between physical disability and evil (for example, Captain Hook) or horror (for example, Frankenstein) serves as a major method by which cultural stereotypes are reinforced and transmitted (cf. Bogdan *et al.* 1982).

7 The importance of personal social integration valued social participation, especially for people at risk of social devaluation

As noted above, Wolfensberger's reformulation of normalisation places at its centre a strong emphasis on the integration of devalued individuals into the wider society. As Wolfensberger and Thomas indicate

> normalization requires that, to the highest degree and in as many areas of life as feasible, a (devalued) person or group have the opportunity to be personally integrated into the valued life of society. This means that as much as possible, (devalued) people would be enabled to: live in normative housing within the valued community, and with (not just near to) valued people; be educated with their non-devalued peers; work in the same facilities as ordinary people; and be involved in a positive fashion in worship, recreation, shopping, and all the other activities in which members of society engage.
>
> (Wolfensberger and Thomas 1983: 27)

The importance of integration arises from two related concerns: the need to provide optimal conditions under which devalued individuals can acquire (through imitation and the exposure to normative role expectancies) socially valued characteristics; and the need to provide the conditions by which social stereotypes can be challenged by direct experience.

These successive reformulations of the principle of normalisation have been elaborated through the development of a series of evaluation materials whose primary use lies in assessing the extent to which services implement the principle of normalisation (Wolfensberger and Glenn 1973a, 1973b, 1975a, 1975b; Wolfensberger and Thomas 1983). The specific implications of the North American version of normalisation are defined in considerable detail in the latest of these evaluation instruments, Program Analysis of Service Systems Implementation of Normalization Goals, more commonly referred to as PASSING (Wolfensberger and Thomas 1983). The development of PASSING and its related evaluation tool Program Analysis of Service Systems (PASS) are presented in detail elsewhere (see Lindley and Wainwright, this volume); nevertheless, PASSING is recounted here in order to explain more fully the content of normalisation.

PROGRAM ANALYSIS OF SERVICES SYSTEMS IMPLEMENTATION OF NORMALISATION GOALS (PASSING)

PASSING consists of a forty-two item rating scale designed for use by a team of three or more trained evaluators to assess the extent to which a human service reflects the principle of normalisation in its organisation and operation (Wolfensberger 1983b). The items are divided into two main categories: those which are primarily related to the impact of the service on the *social image* of service users, and items which are primarily related to the impact of the service on their *personal competency*. These two main categories are further broken down into subsections which focus upon: the physical setting of the service; ways in which the service groups people together and supports relationships between people; and ways in which the service structures people's activities.

Table 1.1 summarises the types of questions each subsection asks of a service and indicates how each subsection contributes to the overall assessment of the service.

Table 1.1 Summary of structure and examples of content of PASSING
(Wolfensberger and Thomas 1983)

Impact of the service on the social image of service
  users: (27 items, 51 per cent of total score)

The Physical Setting of the Service (11 ratings, 17 per cent total)
  Does the service blend in with the neighbourhood in which it is located? Is it
  attractive? Does the appearance of the service match its use (for example, if
  the service is primarily a home for people, does it look like the type of place
  valued people would have as a home)? Does the setting portray its users as
  being younger or older than they actually are? Does the location or history of
  the service result in its users being associated with valued, neutral or devalued
  images or activities?

User Groupings and Relationships in the Service (7 ratings, 15 per cent total)
  Is the service located in close proximity to other services for people at risk of
  devaluation? Does the service congregate people with dissimilar devaluing
  characteristics on the same site? Can the numbers of users served on the site
  be accommodated by the available ordinary resources in the local community?
  Does the service support its users in participating in valued activities, in
  valued settings with valued citizens? Are service workers valued citizens in
  their own right?

User Activities and Use of Time (3 ratings, 8 per cent total)
  Do the activities in which users participate and their allocation of time to
  different activities enhance or diminish their social image? Are the various
  functions which the programme serves (for example, residential, vocational)
  separated in time and space in culturally typical ways? Are users rights
  promoted and safeguarded?

Miscellaneous (6 ratings, 11 per cent total)
  Does the programme support users to portray themselves in a positive
  manner? Does the service support users to own possessions that will enhance
  their social standing? Do service workers talk to and about users in respectful
  ways? Is the source of funding and names associated with the service
  enhancing or demeaning to service users?

Impact of the service on the competence of service users:
  (15 ratings, 49 per cent of total score)

The Physical Setting of the Service (6 ratings, 16 per cent total)
  Is the service accessible to users, their families and the public? Is the service
  located in close proximity to ordinary resources within the community which
  can act as settings for positive contact between users and valued citizens? Is
  the setting comfortable? Does the setting incorporate responsible levels of
  challenge to users? Does it avoid over- and underprotection? Does the
  physical structure of the setting support the development of users' individual
  identities?

User Grouping and Relationships in the Service (6 ratings, 22 per cent total)
  Does the size and composition of groupings of users within the service

provide the optimal conditions for users to acquire valued characteristics? Does the service support its users in participating in valued activities, in valued settings with valued citizens? What is the quality of interactions between and among workers, users and the public? Does the service support the development of users' individual identities and self-expression? Does the service support the users in developing a culturally valued socio-sexual identity?

User Activities and Use of Time (3 ratings, 11 per cent total)
Does the substantive content of the programme address the most important needs of the service users? Are users supported in using their time in the most effective way possible in order to enhance their competencies? Does the service support users in owning possessions which will enhance their abilities?

Wolfensberger's successive reformulations and relabelling of normalisation differ from the earlier Scandinavian approaches in several major aspects: Wolfensberger has explicitly attempted to develop normalisation into a seemingly scientific social theory; Wolfensberger views the fundamental aims of normalisation in terms of changing the status of social groupings; and Wolfensberger's 'theory' of normalisation is purportedly applicable to any social group who are devalued or at risk of devaluation in any society.

Wolfensberger's reformulation of normalisation changed its basic nature from an egalitarian imperative to a *theory* regarding the modification of the social status of deviant groups. Indeed, Wolfensberger has stated that

normalization, and even more since its reformulation as social role valorization, . . . is . . . a theoretical system, grounded deeply and broadly in social and behavioral science, in which there are really very few bits and pieces that do not have extensive empirical support.

(Wolfensberger 1989: 181)

As noted above this transformation was achieved by basing normalisation on then fashionable societal reaction theories of deviance. Indeed, normalisation itself has been described as an 'augmented application of societal reaction theory' (Burton 1983: 55). It is interesting to note, therefore, that societal reaction theories have now largely been abandoned by sociologists as their rather romantic portrayal of members of all deviant groups as being the poor victims of society was questionable. Also, they failed to generate either significant empirical research in support of their propositions or to provide a coherent historical analysis of changes in social reactions to deviance, within the context of the larger social system (cf. Scull 1984a, 1984b). These two later criticisms are particularly relevant to normalisation (or social role valorization) as a theory.

Normalisation proponents have to date been notably reluctant to examine critically specific propositions contained within the theory. Whilst there is insufficient space here to review the empirical foundations of normalisation, it is worth noting that most of the specific propositions contained in normalisation have not been adequately evaluated against an appropriate range of outcomes and the evidence which does exist is often equivocal (for example, Eyman *et al.* 1979, 1987). The use of the theoretical perspectives underpinning normalisation to explain social (for example, Wolfensberger 1987) or historical (for example, Wolfensberger 1975) processes leads, as a result of its emphasis upon the role of ideology, 'into moralism, situating the problem in the minds and hearts of people, rather than in the relations between them' (Burton 1983: 65). Indeed, Wolfensberger's notion of social intent represents the type of 'anthropomorphic conspiracy theory' (Rock 1974: 144) characteristic of the failings of societal reaction theory in this area.

Wolfensberger's social theory of normalisation provides a blueprint for human services which assists them in contributing toward the revaluation of deviant groups. While the revaluation of disadvantaged groups is likely to lead to improvements in the quality of life of group members, Wolfensberger's version of normalisation seeks to reverse or safeguard against the basic social processes that result in deviance. A consequence of this broader objective is that issues of immediate relevance to the quality of life of disabled or disadvantaged people (for example, personal well-being or happiness, the expression of individual choice) become secondary to the social status of the devalued or disadvantaged group as a whole. For example, Wolfensberger discusses the dilemma presented to normalisation advocates when a devalued person chooses a devalued option, thus:

> first, one pursues the line of persuasion, pedagogy, modelling and other forms of culturally normative social influences to steer a person toward a course of action one desires. Second, one imposes coercion only where one would do so legally in the larger societal context, i.e. where one would do so with other (valued) citizens of the same age. Third, one chooses the least restrictive alternative if one does coerce.
>
> (Wolfensberger 1980a: 110)

Interestingly, he includes in options for non-coercive change 'systematic and long term reinforcement for emitting the desired responses' (Wolfensberger 1980a: 110). For Wolfensberger 'the right not to be segregated and institutionalised . . . is really a bigger issue than the restriction of individual choice' (Wolfensberger 1980a: 93). This is, of course, in marked contrast to the earlier Scandinavian definitions where the basic human and civil rights of the *individual* provided the foundation for action. In fact, Perrin and Nirje strongly criticise Wolfensberger for 'specifying various standards of behaviour to which a mentally handicapped person must conform' and conclude that 'this authoritarian approach, however benevolent in its intentions, represents an unwarranted abuse of the powers of the therapeutic state' (Perrin and Nirje 1985: 71).

Wolfensberger reformulated normalisation in such a way as to make it applicable to any deviant group within any society, or indeed, to any group at risk of being devalued. Broadening the scope of the concept to such an extent indicates that he considered the programme of action advocated by normalisation as equally applicable to ethnic or cultural minorities, women and other oppressed or disadvantaged classes. While the theory *could* be applied to such a range of groups, the strategy which it advocates for bringing about social change is one which many members of minority groups would find unacceptable, that is, the adoption by them of the roles, culture and expectations of the dominant group. Such a process could be expected to lead to the destruction of minority cultures (although of course, women are not a minority) and argues against the organisation of consciousness raising or self-help groups as a tactic for change (cf. Szivos and Travers 1988; Szivos, this volume).

NORMALISATION IN THE UK: O'BRIEN'S SERVICE ACCOMPLISHMENTS

The introduction of normalisation to the UK has, in many ways, followed the sequence of developments and influences outlined above. Following the series of inquiries into conditions in long stay institutions during the late 1960s and 1970s, the Scandinavian formulations of normalisation were influential in terms of shaping ideas on the design of new services and the remodelling of old institutions for people with learning difficulties (for example, Centre on Environment for the Handicapped 1972; Gunzberg 1970; Gunzberg and Gunzberg 1973; Nirje 1970).

Over the past decade, however, Wolfensberger's formulation of the principle of normalisation has become dominant through sustained advocacy by the Campaign for People with Mental Handicaps (for example, Campaign for Mentally Handicapped People 1984; O'Brien and Lyle 1983; O'Brien and Tyne 1981; Thomas *et al.* 1978; Wertheimer 1985), the Community and Mental Handicap Education and Research Association (Tyne 1987), the King's Fund Centre (Blunden and Allen 1987; King's Fund Centre 1980, 1984; Towell 1988) and the Independent Development Council for People with Mental Handicap (Independent Development Council for People with Mental Handicap 1986).

Throughout this period, the interpretation of normalisation provided by O'Brien (for example, O'Brien 1980, 1985, 1987; O'Brien and Lyle 1983;

O'Brien and Tyne 1981) has come to be particularly influential. While not presenting a new definition or theoretical formulation, O'Brien has drawn out the implications of normalisation in terms of what services should try to achieve or accomplish for users. He identifies five major service accomplishments.

1 Ensuring that service users are *present* in the community by supporting their actual physical presence in the same neighbourhoods, schools, work places, shops, recreation facilities and churches as ordinary citizens.

2 Ensuring that service users are supported in *making choices* about their lives by encouraging people to understand their situation, the options they face and to act in their own interest both in small everyday matters and in such important issues as who to live with and what type of work to do.

3 Developing the *competence* of service users by developing skills and attributes that are functional and meaningful in natural community environments and relationships, i.e. skills and attributes which significantly decrease a person's dependency or develop personal characteristics that other people value.

4 Enhancing the *respect* afforded to service users by developing and maintaining a positive reputation for people who use the service by ensuring that the choice of activities, locations, forms of dress and use of language promote the perception of people with disabilities as developing citizens.

5 Ensuring that service users *participate* in the life of the community by supporting people's natural relationships with their families, neighbours and co-workers and, when necessary, widening each individual's network of personal relationships to include an increasing number of people.

The differences between Wolfensberger and O'Brien are of emphasis and style rather than of theory. While not explicitly rejecting Wolfensberger's theoretical formulations, O'Brien's notions of service accomplishments are devoid of the sociological trappings of Wolfensberger's theory. They place major emphasis upon delineating the implications of normalisation in terms of the lifestyle or quality of life of members of the devalued group and return individual choice to a central position in normalisation. As such, O'Brien's interpretation of normalisation can be seen to represent a return to the values underpinning the initial conceptions of normalisation and a retreat from the grand theorising of Wolfensberger.

CONCLUSIONS

Normalisation and social role valorization are likely to remain influential concepts in the continuing debates about the most effective ways of structuring services for people with disabilities. Such influence does not, of course, automatically translate into changes in actual practice. Indeed, Wolfensberger summarises the situation thus:

> Contrary to common claims, few human services have really embraced social role valorization, or are likely to do so. If the rhetoric about it is an ocean, then its committed implementation is a drizzle, and even that often turns into a frizzle.
>
> (Wolfensberger 1989: 184)

The intention behind this attempt to clarify the different meanings of the term(s) normalisation and to point out some of the key similarities and differences is to guide practice more effectively. Hopefully, increasing clarity in the conceptual debate will have an impact on the quality of services provided to people with disabilities who may need long-term support.

REFERENCES

Anninson, J.E., and Young, W.H.L. (1980) 'The future forms of residential services for mentally retarded people in Australia – a delphi study', *Australian and New Zealand Journal of Developmental Disabilities* 6: 167–80.

Bank-Mikkelsen, N. (1980) 'Denmark', in R.J. Flynn and K.E. Nitsch (eds) *Normalisation, Social Integration and Community Services*, Austin, Texas: Pro-Ed.

Blunden, R., and Allen, D. (1987) *Facing the Challenge: An ordinary life for people with learning difficulties and challenging behaviours*, London: King's Fund.

Bogdan, R., Biklen, D., Shapiro, A., and Spelkoman, D. (1982) 'The disabled: Media's monster', *Social Policy* 12: 32–5.

Brown, P. (1985) *The Transfer of Care: Psychiatric deinstitutionalization and its aftermath*, London: Routledge and Kegan Paul.

Burton, M. (1983) 'Understanding mental health services: Theory and practice', *Critical Social Policy* 7: 54–74.

Campaign for Mentally Handicapped People (1984) *Hope for the Future? CMH's evidence to the Social Services Committee on community care*, London: Campaign for Mentally Handicapped People.

Castellani, P.J. (1987) *The Political Economy of Developmental Disabilities*, Baltimore: Paul H. Brookes.

Centre on Environment for the Handicapped (1972) *Room for Improvement: A better environment for the mentally handicapped*, London: King's Fund Centre.

Davies, N.J. (1975) *Sociological Constructions of Deviance*, Dubuque, Iowa: Brown.

Eyman, R.K., Borthwick-Duffy, S.A., and Sheehy, N.L. (1987) 'A longitudinal study of foster care placement', in S. Landesman and P. Vietze (eds) *Living Environments and Mental Retardation*, Washington, DC: American Association on Mental Retardation.

Eyman, R.K., Demaine, G.C., and Lei, T. (1979) 'Relationship between community environments and resident changes in adaptive behavior', *American Journal of Mental Deficiency* 83: 330–8.

Grunewald, K. (1986) 'The intellectually handicapped in Sweden – new legislation in a bid for normalisation', *Current Sweden* 345: 1–10.

Gunzberg, H.C. (1970) 'The hospital as a normalizing training environment', *Journal of Mental Subnormality* 16: 71–83.

Gunzberg, H.C., and Gunzberg, A.L. (1973) *Mental Handicap and Physical Environment*, London: Balliere Tindall.

Independent Development Council for People with Mental Handicap (1986) *Pursuing Quality*, London: Independent Development Council.

King's Fund Centre (1980) *An Ordinary Life: Comprehensive locally-based residential services for mentally handicapped people*, London: King's Fund Centre.

King's Fund Centre (1984) *An Ordinary Working Life: Vocational services for people with mental handicap*, London: King's Fund Centre.

Lemert, E. (1967) *Human Deviance, Social Problems and Social Control*, New Jersey: Prentice-Hall.

McCarver, R.B., and Cavalier, A.R. (1983) 'Philosophical concepts and attitudes underlying programming for the mentally retarded', in J.L. Matson and F. Andrasik (eds) *Treatment Issues and Innovations in Mental Retardation*, London: Plenum.

Nirje, B. (1969) 'The normalization principle and its human management implications', in R.B. Kugel and W. Wolfensberger (eds) *Changing Patterns in Residential Services for the Mentally Retarded*, Washington, DC: Presidential Committee on Mental Retardation.

Nirje, B. (1970) 'The normalization principle – implications and comments', *Journal of Mental Subnormality* 16: 62–70.

Nirje, B. (1972) 'The right to self-determination', in W. Wolfensberger (ed.) *The Principle of Normalization in Human Services*, Toronto: National Institute on Mental Retardation.

Nirje, B. (1980) 'The normalization principle', in R.J. Flynn and K.E. Nitsch (eds) *Normalization, Social Integration and Community Services*, Baltimore: University Park Press.

Nirje, B. (1985) 'The basis and logic of the normalization principle', *Australian and New Zealand Journal of Developmental Disabilities* 11: 65–8.

O'Brien, J. (1980) 'The principle of normalization: A foundation for effective services', in J.F. Gardner, L. Long, R. Nichols and D.M. Iagulli (eds) *Program Issues in Developmental Disabilities: A resource manual for surveyors and reviewers*, Baltimore: Paul H. Brookes.

O'Brien, J. (1985) *Normalization Training Through PASS 3: Team Leader Manual*, Decature, GA: Responsive Systems Associates.

O'Brien, J. (1987) 'A guide to life style planning: Using The Activities Catalogue to integrate services and natural support systems', in B.W. Wilcox and G.T. Bellamy (eds) *The Activities Catalogue: An alternative curriculum for youth and adults with severe disabilities*, Baltimore: Brookes.

O'Brien, J. and Lyle, C. (1983) *Planning Spaces: A manual for anyone who helps set up human service facilities*, London: The Campaign for Mentally Handicapped People.

O'Brien, J. and Tyne, A. (1981) *The Principle of Normalisation: A foundation for effective services*, London: The Campaign for Mentally Handicapped People.

Pelletier, J., and Richler, D. (1982) *Major Issues in Community Living for Mentally Handicapped Persons: Reflections on the Canadian experience*, Toronto: National Institute on Mental Retardation.

Perrin, B., and Nirje, B. (1985) 'Setting the record straight: A critique of some frequent misconceptions of the normalization principle', *Australian and New Zealand Journal of Developmental Disabilities* 11: 69–74.

Rock, P. (1974) 'The sociology of deviancy and conceptions of moral order', *British Journal of Criminology* 14: 139–49.

Scheerenberger, R.C. (1983) *A History of Mental Retardation*, Baltimore: P.H. Brookes.

Scull, A.T. (1984a) 'Competing perspectives on deviance', *Deviant Behavior* 5: 275–89.

Scull, A.T. (1984b) *Decarceration: Community treatment of the deviant – a radical view* (2nd Edition), Cambridge: University Press.

Szivos, S.E., and Travers, E. (1988) 'Consciousness raising among mentally handicapped people: A critique of the implications of normalization', *Human Relations* 41: 641–53.

Thomas, D., Firth, H., and Kendall, A. (1978) *ENCOR – A way ahead*, London: Campaign for Mentally Handicapped People.

Towell, D. (1988) *An Ordinary Life in Practice*, London: King's Fund Centre.

Tyne, A. (1987) 'Shaping community services: The impact of an idea', in N. Malin (ed.) *Reassessing Community Care*, Beckenham, Kent: Croom Helm.

Tyne, A. (1989) 'Normalisation: The next steps', *Community Living* 3: 7–8.

Wertheimer, A. (1985) *Going to Work*, London: The Campaign for People with Mental Handicaps.

Wolfensberger, W. (1972) *The Principle of Normalization in Human Services*, Toronto: National Institute on Mental Retardation.

Wolfensberger, W. (1975) *The Origin and Nature of our Institutional Models*, Syracuse: Human Policy Press.

Wolfensberger, W. (1980a) 'The definition of normalisation: Update, problems, disagreements and misunderstandings', in R.J. Flynn and K.E. Nitsch (eds) *Normalization, Social Integration and Community Services*, Baltimore: University Park Press.

Wolfensberger, W. (1980b) 'A brief overview of the principle of normalisation', in R.J. Flynn and K.E. Nitsch (eds) *Normalization, Social Integration and Community Services*, Baltimore: University Park Press.

Wolfensberger, W. (1983a) 'Social role valorization: A proposed new term for the principal of normalization', *Mental Retardation* 21: 234–9.

Wolfensberger, W. (1983b) *Guidelines for Evaluators During a PASS, PASSING or Similar Assessment of Human Service Quality*, Toronto: NIMR.

Wolfensberger, W. (1984) 'A reconceptualization of normalization as social role valorization', *Mental Retardation* (Canadian) 34: 22–5.

Wolfensberger, W. (1987) 'Values in the funding of social services', *American Journal of Mental Deficiency* 92: 141–3.

Wolfensberger, W. (1989) 'Self-injurious behavior, behavioristic responses, and social role valorization: A reply to Mulick and Kedesdy', *Mental Retardation* 27: 181–4.

Wolfensberger, W., and Glenn, S. (1973a) *Program Analysis of Service Systems*, Vol. I. Handbook (2nd Edition), Toronto: National Institute on Mental Retardation.

LOTHIAN COLLEGE OF HEALTH STUDIES LIBRARY

Wolfensberger, W., and Glenn, S. (1973b) *Program Analysis of Service Systems*, Vol. II. Field Manual, Toronto: National Institute on Mental Retardation.

Wolfensberger, W., and Glenn, S. (1975a) *PASS 3: Program Analysis of Service Systems*, Handbook (3rd Edition), Toronto: National Institute on Mental Retardation.

Wolfensberger, W., and Glenn, S. (1975b) *PASS 3: Program Analysis of Service Systems*, Field Manual, Toronto: National Institute on Mental Retardation.

Wolfensberger, W., and Thomas, S. (1983) *PASSING: Program Analysis of Service Systems Implementation of Normalization Goals*, Toronto: National Institute on Mental Retardation.

Wolfensberger, W., and Tullman, S. (1982) 'A brief outline of the principle of normalization', *Rehabilitation Psychology* 27: 131–45.

2 Normalisation training
Conversion or commitment?

Peter Lindley and Tony Wainwright

This chapter provides an overview of normalisation training and its developments, both internationally and in the United Kingdom. It describes the history and development of training, different forms of training available and considers the impact of training on individuals and on services generally. It will also present some of the more recent ideas which have emerged from the Training Institute for Human Service Planning and Change Agentry at Syracuse University, led by Professor Wolfensberger. These address the moral dimension of human service work and have been presented in a number of workshops including 'Threats to the Sanctity of Life of Handicapped and Afflicted People' (Wolfensberger 1987a) and 'How to Function with Personal Moral Coherency in a Disfunctional (Human Service) World' (Wolfensberger 1987b).

The most common form of normalisation training has taken place in Program Analysis of Service Systems (PASS) workshops (Wolfensberger and Glenn 1973, 1975) or Program Analysis of Service Systems Implementation of Normalization Goals (PASSING) workshops (Wolfensberger and Thomas 1983). These workshops were introduced into this country by a small group of committed individuals, who have had a definitive and positive influence on the British development of the normalisation philosophy.

The workshops have been popular with sponsors and participants and the networks which emerged maintained a powerful momentum for service change. Nevertheless, there was considerable criticism of the manner in which the teaching was conducted. Most of the criticism focused on a debate about the dynamics within the workshops, leading people to question whether the teaching methods constituted indoctrination, or provided a powerful emotional window on the lives of people who depend on services, lives which were often distressingly deprived. The literature on normalisation training tends to be polemical. It either strongly advocates the status quo in PASS/ING training (Wolfensberger 1978, 1983, 1984,

1985; O'Brien and Tyne 1981; Tyne 1989) or is strongly critical (Baldwin 1985; Clifford 1987). This chapter aims to give a balanced view of the benefits and the problems of normalisation training and traces the development of more recent training concerning the moral nature of human service work.

THE HISTORY OF NORMALISATION TRAINING

Normalisation workshops started in the United States in the late 1960s. The PASS framework was developed by Wolfensberger around that time to fulfil four purposes:

- to establish a standard for normalising human management agency performance;
- to provide an objective means of assessing (either by internal or external evaluation) the quality of the human service, thereby to assess quality change over time and compare the performance of different services;
- to provide a rational means for allocating limited funds on a competitive basis;
- to function as a teaching tool for disseminating the normalisation principle.

(Wolfensberger 1972: 226)

The third purpose was actually the one that furnished the strongest initial impetus for the development of PASS. In 1969, the Nebraska Legislature enacted a mental retardation community services bill that provided financial state matching for local programmes. However, the initial allocation was so modest that a way had to be found to disperse the money through a process that would be unaffected by political and other pressures and in such a fashion as to make maximal impact. PASS was at this stage a relatively crude instrument which was used to judge applications for funding (Wolfensberger 1972; Wolfensberger and Glenn 1973). This initial evaluation instrument was then developed further and was eventually published as PASS but referred to as PASS 2. The numbering of the different editions of PASS is somewhat confusing, PASS 1 was never published and the first published version was in fact a second edition (Wolfensberger and Glenn 1973). Having refined these instruments, the Training Institute at Syracuse University remained the major centre for the development and dissemination of the materials.

From its inception, people using PASS as an evaluation instrument were required to participate in a training programme. It was regarded as an important part of the standardisation process that raters become familiar with the basis on which the ratings were derived, much as skilled users of any measuring instrument are required to undergo uniform training. Although there have been variations, the pattern of training remains essentially as it was conceived at that time.

From its initial focus on the training of evaluators, PASS has moved on to become the basis for extensive training programmes for service workers. The ideas have gained international acceptance (Cocks 1988; Emerson, this volume; Tyne 1989). In Australia, for example, the Training and Evaluation for Change Association was inaugurated in 1988. It maintains close links with the Training Institute at Syracuse University and a number of its key members attended the Institute's training. The Association aims to increase the number of training leaders, develop a range of training events and support a small number of people to become trainers at an advanced level. The major focus of its activities has been to conduct training events for members and others and to increase their understanding of normalisation and social role valorisation. Similar developments have occurred in other countries and the materials, together with the field manuals, have been translated into a number of languages, including French, Spanish, Norwegian and Welsh.

THE ARRIVAL OF PASS IN BRITAIN

In parallel with developments elsewhere, the Community and Mental Handicap Educational and Research Association (CMHERA) – an organisation set up to promote the interests of people with learning difficulties through training and research – has been largely responsible for the successful development of normalisation training in Britain. A measure of their success is the continuing demand for training and the outstanding popularity of the training approach. PASS/ING training began here in 1978 when Alan Tyne, having attended a PASS workshop in the United States, subsequently invited a senior trainer (Joe Osborn) from Syracuse to run a normalisation workshop in Britain. This led directly to an invitation to John O'Brien and Connie Lyle, at that time colleagues of Wolfensberger, to lead a further PASS workshop in 1980. Between 1980 and 1982 they ran a number of small workshops. The first independent British workshop, run by Paul Williams and Alan Tyne, took place in 1982. It was intended that this would begin a process of developing national interest in normalisation training and in the use of PASS as an evaluation tool in Britain. By 1989, over 3000 people had attended PASS workshops organised by CMHERA.

The introduction of PASSING (Wolfensberger and Thomas 1983) followed an invitation from CMHERA to Susan Thomas, co-author of PASSING, to lead a PASSING workshop in 1984. Subsequently,

PASSING workshops have been more frequently run and, together with PASS, are the main vehicles for the teaching of normalisation and/or social role valorisation in this country. Throughout this process of growth, those responsible for normalisation training in Britain have retained close links with the Institute at Syracuse.

THE FORMAT AND CONTENT OF NORMALISATION TRAINING

The 1975 Handbook to the PASS 3 rating system offers clear guidelines for how training should be conducted:

> Ideally, an introductory training session should be six days long, and should involve field visits on the third and fifth days. The fourth day would be devoted to writing a report on the experiences of the third day . . .
>
> (Wolfensberger and Thomas 1983: 71)

The handbook outlines a schedule for a typical introductory PASS workshop and, although the emphasis during training has changed substantially, this format has remained essentially the same.

It is not the purpose of this chapter to give a detailed description of the two instruments and readers are referred to the original publications (Wolfensberger and Glenn 1975; Wolfensberger and Thomas 1983). However, a summary is provided here of the organisation of the rating system. PASS identifies fifty independent dimensions of service quality (see PASS 3 Field Manual, Wolfensberger and Glenn 1975). They represent an attempt to distil from the normalisation principle a set of standards against which services can be judged. The fifty ratings are divided into a number of clusters. There are fourteen ratings on physical and social integration. These ratings 'refer to those measures and practices which maximise a person's (potential) participation in the mainstream of the culture' (ibid.: 1). There are twelve ratings on age and cultural appropriateness. This area is covered by 'seven ratings which affect the way a person is perceived in relation to his chronological age' and an additional five ratings relating to issues of common customs and perceptions (ibid.: 31). The rating of model coherency is

> concerned with whether a number of variables within a program combine harmoniously so as to meet the specific needs of each client at that particular time of his life.
>
> (Wolfensberger and Glenn 1975: 35)

Three ratings reflect an orientation to developmental growth and a further four ratings deal with the concept of quality of setting, which includes physical comfort, environmental beauty, individualisation and the quality of interpersonal interactions. The remaining sixteen ratings are concerned with administration and management.

The structure of PASSING has many similarities. The forty-two ratings are divided into two broad categories: twenty-seven of them relate primarily to the impact of the service on the social image of the client and the remaining fifteen to the impact of the service on their competence. The image enhancement ratings are grouped into four main areas – physical setting, the way people are grouped by the service, the activities provided to clients and the language and labels used to describe them. These concern the extent to which the service practices enhance or damage the social image of the clients. Competency enhancement ratings assess three broad issues – first, the extent to which the physical setting of the service is able to enhance the competency of the clients; second, the ways in which people are grouped together in terms of maximising their potential to learn; finally, the way the service structures activities and time and the consequences of this for learning (Wolfensberger and Thomas 1983).

The majority of PASS/ING workshops in Britain are used to provide an introduction to normalisation and rarely to teach either of the instruments as evaluation tools. The workshops are intensive residential events. In the information packs sent to participants beforehand they are advised that there will be no time for anything other than the business of the workshop. The rationale for this intensity is to help participants make space for a fresh perspective. We are all constantly exposed to the conventional wisdom underpinning human services which maintains that services are as they are because of the characteristics of the people who rely on them, rather than the unconscious social processes that devalue clients. Since the workshops are to provide an opportunity for learning about normalisation, participants are asked to suspend their preconceptions and use the assumptions and principles of normalisation to consider the ways in which services are organised. This process needs careful management as it can sometimes result in the participants feeling that they are being subjected to ways of learning akin to 'brain washing' (see for example Clifford 1986 and Wainwright 1986 for an alternative point of view).

The workshops aim to formulate an accurate description of a service, both rooted in and accountable to the experiences of the people who depend on it. Each team visits a different service and at the end of the workshop gives constructive feedback to the managers. Participants are encouraged to suspend judgement, not to ask *why* things are as they are, but to describe as accurately as possible what is taking place.

If weaknesses were accepted because of endless why's with which they are often excused or explained, PASS would be a dishonest system and PASS scores would cease to be comparable across services. It is a principle which many people find difficult to internalise. We are brought up to be 'nice'; we excuse weaknesses in human beings and in human services; we shy away from any 'mechanistic' determination of quality.

(Wolfensberger and Glenn 1975: 30)

This process allows participants to be sensitised to the lives of people with disabilities. Participants are encouraged to take a systemic view, that is, to focus on how the service works as a system of many interrelated parts, and so avoid blaming individual workers.

The workshop lasts for five or six days. The first half of the workshop is spent learning about normalisation through presentations on social devaluation and on the common experiences of people with disabilities. The seven core themes are explained (see Emerson, this volume). A brief introduction is given to each of the ratings. The participants also work in teams, focusing on the application of the ratings to simulations of three different services. The remainder of the workshop is devoted to applying the ratings to an actual service. The participants, in teams of six to eight with a team leader, visit a service and collect information in order to complete each of the ratings in the manual. The most important method for gathering this information is for each participant to get to know an individual who uses the service. This is explicitly to learn about the person as one human being to another and for a short while to enter into their lives.

Getting to know a service user in this way can be a powerful experience and has been described by one participant as 'similar to visiting starving people in a third world country, except that the people live in our own land'. This aspect of the workshop, more than any other, provokes extreme reactions, both positive and negative. On the positive side, people report that they have learned more from that one brief meeting than from all their professional training about the lives of people with disabilities. On the negative side, there are often strong feelings that the team has intruded on the privacy and emotional life of the people using the service, sometimes without their consent (despite the efforts of the workshop organisers) and in a way that apparently negates the very principles which the workshop aims to teach.

On the last day the team leader gives verbal feedback on the team's findings to the service managers and users, who are encouraged to tape record the session for people who are unable to attend. The workshop finishes following a plenary forum, where participants share their learning and give feedback to the other teams, without disclosing details which would identify the services they have visited.

THE ROLE OF TEAM LEADERS

The role of the team leader is central to the success of the workshops. Team leaders organise the learning of the team, supervise the reading assignments, lead the team through the slide simulations and help the team to process information from the presentations. They manage all aspects of the practice evaluation, including the timetable for the site visits, making sure that each participant carries out the required assignments. Team leaders conduct an extensive interview with the service manager and facilitate the conciliation of the ratings. Finally they prepare and deliver the feedback.

Keeping the team focused at each stage of the workshop is an important task. Participants learning about normalisation and the ratings in PASS/ING are presented with new and strongly value-laden information, which is necessarily challenging to their assumptions and beliefs. In visiting the site and meeting the people who work and/or live there, participants concentrate on the 'whats' rather than the 'whys'. In rating the service, teams may be tempted to compromise because of concerns about how they are going to deliver their findings to staff: it is the team leaders task to help the group focus on the hard evidence collected during the site visit and to rate the service accurately, purely on that material. Teams frequently conclude that the service provided does not, at least in normalisation terms, reach a sufficiently high standard to ensure a reasonable quality of life for service users.

The intensity and the structure of the workshops create powerful group dynamics, which can either facilitate or impede the group task. The management of these dynamics is complex and fundamentally problematic. The central task of the team leader is to ensure that participants gain insights which are rooted in genuine contact with the realities of human services rather than from the feelings created through being a member of the group. The material is often personally challenging and contentious and the discussion usually continues until the early hours of the morning in order to finish the ratings. Not all team leaders are skilled in managing this process and many get caught up in it themselves. An unskilled team leader may fail to keep the emotional focus on the service and so allow the internal group dynamics to take over. Participants are also being asked to accept an implicit values-base with which they may not be able explicitly to articulate disagreement. These tensions have been the source of some of the criticisms that have described the experience of a PASS workshop as 'quasi-religious'.

Because of these inherent conflicts, team leaders are placed in a demanding and difficult role. Regrettably, many that we have spoken to, and indeed worked with, have expressed concern at the lack of training and support available to them and many only lead a team once or twice. Despite this, there are a number of people eager to continue team leading.

The style of the workshop and its management were initially prescribed by Wolfensberger in considerable detail. The Standard Operating Procedures or SOPs are imbued with a legendary character as they provide instructions on how to ensure the workshop is properly conducted, despite the uncertainty of the real world. There is great emphasis on high standards in training, which involves conforming to the methods and using the materials developed by the Training Institute. The emphasis comes from Wolfensberger's not unreasonable belief that the ideas in normalisation can be easily misunderstood, become corrupted, and used for rather unsavoury ends. An example of this is the way normalisation rhetoric is used to justify the most gross abuses of handicapped people.

> Of course, perversions of normalisation occur everywhere, including in connection with community services. For instance one mental health administrator in New York said 'community mental health is normalisation'. Somebody else said that normalization means that, if necessary, one uses violence to make non-normal people normal, or at least to make them act in acceptable ways.
>
> (Wolfensberger 1980: 104)

There are differences in the workshop format in PASS/ING training between Britain and the United States. In the United States, there are two site visits and no verbal feedback to the site. Detailed written evaluations are prepared by either a team leader or delegated assistant, which is checked by a senior trainer before being submitted to the site. This process may take months. In Britain, verbal feedback is given by the team leader to the site on the last day of the workshop. This can provoke strong disquiet among participants who may be tired and angry at what they have seen. If the team leader is also tired, angry and/or unskilled, the resulting feedback can make service providers feel that they are being attacked and blamed for the inadequacies of the service.

THE IMPACT OF NORMALISATION TRAINING

Most (if not all) services for people with learning difficulties claim to have based their service developments on normalisation. More recently, the principle has been extended to services for people with mental health problems and services for elderly people. It is an issue of some importance as to whether any of these services have, in fact, implemented normalisation, or simply incorporated it into their rhetoric. Nevertheless, the growth in the use of the term is due almost solely to the intensive efforts of those involved in the training. The widespread acceptance of the term might also be accounted for by a coincidence of political and social agendas between those who wished to legitimise the closure of large institutions (now widely acknowledged to be a cost-saving venture) and those who were genuinely committed to developing better lives for people with disabilities (Hudson 1990). Research is currently underway to examine the extent to which normalisation has really been implemented in disability services (Pilling 1990).

VARIATIONS ON PASS/ING TRAINING

A number of variations on the basic PASS and PASSING model have been sporadically available. 'Using PASS in Organisational Change' (Kristiansen and Tyne 1985) is a workshop for participants with an existing knowledge of PASS/ING. This workshop enables participants to evaluate a whole service and to build up a comprehensive picture of the way the different elements of the service operate together. This is to enable participants to consider how PASS can be used to develop an agenda for service change. 'Advanced PASS' is for experienced participants and concentrates on the evaluation and feedback to the service used for the site visit rather than learning the ratings or normalisation theory.

O'Brien and Lyle's 'Framework for Accomplishments' (1989) was developed in order to make explicit the outcomes that an effective service should expect to achieve for people. There are a variety of ways in which the Accomplishments workshops have been carried out (and a varying number of accomplishments). One particular version, 'Transitions Training', focuses on training staff working in services in transition from hospital to community care (Lemmer and Braisby 1990) and on identifying service accomplishments for individual users.

'Citizen Advocacy Programme Evaluation' or CAPE (O'Brien and Wolfensberger 1978) is a system which has a similar structure to PASS and uses a corresponding process for evaluating citizen advocacy programmes. As with normalisation, many so-called advocacy programmes use the rhetoric rather than implement the principles and CAPE allows programmes properly to evaluate whether they are translating their principles into practice.

Normalisation training is being increasingly, albeit partially, introduced into mainstream training courses. It has been incorporated into English National Board training for nurses (RNMH). Various health authorities have produced teaching packs using normalisation in considering issues of service design, quality assurance and deinstitutionalisation (see *Bringing People Back Home*, Brown *et al.* 1986–90). It also forms the basis for much

local induction and continuing training in community residential programmes for people with long-term mental health problems and people
with learning difficulties.

Packs and teaching approaches have been developed which focus on
particular aspects of normalisation such as the 'Lifestyles' packs (Brown
and Alcoe 1986) which are designed to help staff groups explore their own
values and preferences in response to a whole range of living situations and
social circumstances. The group consensus is thus used as a reference point
from which participants can evaluate their own service and target possibilities for positive change. 'Outcomes' (Hoskins 1989) is a pack which
uses a board game to help participants explore O'Brien's five accomplishments (O'Brien 1987). It uses the notion of 'trade-offs', whereby an
intervention may be positive on one dimension but less desirable in regard
to another. Thus, for example, being taught how to use a shopping list in the
local supermarket would score highly for competence but might draw
unwelcome attention to the individual and so score low for respect. These
exercises enable workers to clarify their own assumptions and experiences
(which most directly affect service users) through rehearsing everyday
decisions and dilemmas.

Packs such as these, while making the ideas of normalisation accessible
and translating the terminology into everyday language, have, as Wolfensberger feared, diluted the rigorous analysis contained in PASS/ING. This
has led to a wide range of different (mis)understandings of the principle.

REACTIONS TO PASS/ING TRAINING

A central concept in PASS is that of Model Coherency. The concept can
usefully be applied to the training, as well as to the service evaluation. Thus
participants often question whether the training is itself coherent. Do the
various elements of the training fit together in a way that maximises the
opportunities for learning and does the training address the particular needs
of the participants? A major problem here has been that, due to self-
selection, participants have not been a homogeneous group. They have a
wide variety of experiences and attitudes to services and vary in their initial
receptiveness to the ideas. They range from people who have been
blinkered by long periods of professional training to those who themselves
use services as clients or carers.

Recently, Kristiansen (1988) has tackled this problem by adopting the
Training Institute recommendation which requires that before attending
PASS/ING, participants attend a two or three day introductory normal-
isation/social role valorisation workshop. This serves two functions: it
allows the participants to learn something of the principles on which the

workshop will be based and also introduces them to the emotional challenges they may face in the full workshop. Participants can thus choose
whether to attend or not from a position of more informed consent. However, despite this there are occasional mishaps: these take a variety of forms
of which the following examples are typical.

A feature of the workshops is that they do not provide a bridge for
participants returning to work, so that people may misapply normalisation
with unhelpful consequences for services and individual users and workers.
For example, a service was set up for elderly people with early Alzheimer's
disease who had been in hospital for a few weeks and needed a place to
relearn skills so they could return home. The director of the hospital had
heard of normalisation and felt it would be useful for the staff to be trained
to apply the principles. After attending the workshop, the charge nurse
introduced a scheme in one of the wards and required that the principles of
normalisation be rigidly adhered to. The student nurses were instructed to
refer to themselves as friends whenever they spoke on the phone to other
agencies, on the basis that residents would be stigmatised if it were known
that their appointments were being arranged by nurses. The issue of choice
was also regarded as paramount but addressed in a simplistic way so that
the charge nurse decided that a resident could take a shower unassisted. The
resident collapsed and injured his hip. Accidents happen regardless of the
application of normalisation, but in this case normalisation was 'blamed' as
the cause. This last incident led to a backlash by the service and the charge
nurse was reduced two grades and sent to work on one of the back wards.
The unit itself rejected normalisation and changed the operational policy so
that it would aim to provide an environment resembling a nursing home,
rather than an ordinary home.

Individual workers may also find the insights gained in the workshops
difficult to reconcile with their everyday practice. A social worker having
attended a PASS training workshop felt that his professional training was
quite inadequate to help people experiencing such deprivation. He felt that
the course had deskilled him and he found it so hard to function that the
service in which he worked was deprived of his professional skills for some
time. He eventually resolved the dilemma by rejecting normalisation as
being unrealistic. This example highlights a real problem about how to help
participants cope with the mismatch between what their professional training has taught them to provide and what they come to understand through
PASS/ING about what people really need. Insight which leads workers to
question the relevance of much of their professional work can cause
genuine and painful conflicts, both within individuals, and with colleagues.

Another central criticism of PASS/ING is that it does not adequately
address clients' individual feelings of well-being and happiness. This

criticism was regarded as 'partly correct' by Wolfensberger for the following reasons:

1 . . . it does not purport to be a clinical instrument that measures highly individual personal characteristics and dynamics. Thus it is not orientated to specific individuals, but to groups of clients and particularly to the relationships between the service agency and its clients in general.
2 Personal feelings of well-being and happiness are only partially controllable by agency programme structure. Even under optimal conditions, some persons will be unhappy, and will perhaps quite literally create their own Hell. On the other hand some individuals function with a great deal of serenity under very adverse conditions. About the only thing that one can say is that PASS measures conditions which are generally optimal when considered in relation to clients in general and over the long run.
3 Finally, and very profoundly, it is recognised that the creation of normalised conditions of life does not always imply reduction of stress and discomfort in clients. To the contrary: a sheltered and clearly denormalised setting might find it much easier to create contentment in certain clients, while a normalisation-based structure may be demanding, stressful and at times turbulent. For instance the 'dignity-of-risk' does not always bring happiness.

> *It is one of the explicit and honest implications of the normalisation principle and of PASS that what many people call 'happiness' (and a number of related social-psychological states) may not constitute the highest value in earthly life – at least not if they are bought at the expense of independence, self-sufficiency and respect from others, or if they create devaluing attitudes in the public's mind towards additional individuals who are different. They are especially not worth it when one considers how the devaluing attitudes in the minds of citizens brutalize them and in a sense make them morally self-destructive* [our emphasis].

(Wolfensberger 1975: 31–2)

Despite Wolfensberger's explanation, many people working in services have found it difficult to believe in the efficacy of undertaking an evaluation that does not include subjective feelings or state of mind when evaluating the life experiences of people with disabilities, and normalisation has been criticised on these grounds (see Szivos, this volume).

MORAL COHERENCY

In addition to providing social role valorisation and related training events, the Training Institute's mission 'has to do with reading "the signs of the times" and interpreting their meaning for human services' (Wolfensberger 1990b). This mission is carried out by publishing 'TIPS' (Training Institute Publication Series), a duplicated bi-monthly newsletter, and through the Moral Coherency workshop. This workshop was designed for participants who had been inspired by PASS/ING training but had returned to work only to discover that 'it is no longer possible to produce a comprehensive valid human service system in the USA' (Moral Coherency Workshop, Wolfensberger 1987b). Such participants frequently reported feeling disillusioned and/or depressed and unable to continue in human service work.

The workshop allows participants to examine the negative dynamics of a society which opposes rational and moral goals and to explore the difficulties which await those who pursue such goals. Furthermore, it provides an opportunity for participants to examine their own moral stance and to strengthen their commitment to moral and rational goals, regardless of success in the normal sense of the word. It asserts that success should be gauged by whether the person had acted in a morally valid way, not by the usual yardsticks of whether they had planned within the budget or done some clever piece of research. The Moral Coherency workshop lasts six days and is delivered almost entirely in lectures. There is a strong emphasis on 'universals', that is, processes or outcomes that occur always and everywhere. One major aim of the workshop is to demonstrate that there are indeed universally valid ways of acting, and that there are universal societal processes which act to make some members of a social group 'dis'-abled, even to the point of frankly killing them.

As part of the workshop, 'Threats to the Sanctity of Life of Handicapped and Afflicted People', participants are reminded that handicapped people were murdered by the Nazis (Wolfensberger 1981; Lifton 1986) and that the first gas chambers were in hospitals for the handicapped (Klee 1983; Burleigh 1990). Thus participants identify genocidal phenomena and consider the evidence and support for deathmaking and major dimensions of contemporary deathmaking, including where it is carried out and by whom. Deathmaking is defined as 'Any action or pattern of actions that brings about or hastens the death of any person or group'. The workshop challenges participants to develop a moral stance in confronting deathmaking practices. Not surprisingly many participants strongly disagree with the material and deny that the killing described is actually taking place. Others find themselves challenged in a fundamental way which often leads to a re-examination of the moral basis of their lives.

The Training Institute regards the issue of 'deathmaking' of handicapped and afflicted people as the single most important issue they confront. Much of their current work is aimed at collecting evidence and teaching on this issue. In particular, Wolfensberger singles out abortion and infanticide as the most extensive killing currently practised and also the most 'detoxified'. By this, he means that it is surrounded by euphemism to avoid confronting its true nature. He feels that technological advances have made our society much more 'eugenic' in selecting who will have a life and who will not, and that it is the handicapped who are being selected not to live (Wolfensberger 1987a; Wolfensberger 1990a).

It may seem a long way from the apparently simple notion of normalisation as a way of planning better services for people, to a set of ideas which see services as largely baneful and morally bankrupt. In Wolfensberger's view, the prevailing social attitude is that suffering is a meaningless experience to be avoided at all costs, which results in those in pain being shut away and services playing a significant role in accomplishing this. He considers that life for people with disabilities is not improving and that for the world generally things are looking distinctly gloomy – an unpalatable but plausible notion with which many will identify. In addition, he now teaches workshops specifically for Christians who wish to consider the implications of the Training Institute's work for their faith and practice.

While respecting Wolfensberger's work, O'Brien and many others have been developing strands from the earlier commitment to improving services. The impact of 'Framework for Accomplishments' (O'Brien and Lyle 1989) illustrates the continuing development of workshops and training experiences within this more optimistic tradition.

FUTURE DIRECTIONS

There are conflicting notions on the direction in which normalisation training should proceed in Britain (Williams 1990; Kendrick 1989). These are focused around issues of leadership and standards setting. In particular, there are questions about whether the Training Institute should remain the source of standards for normalisation training in this country or whether the variety of groups loosely organised around CMHERA should continue to develop their own style of training. In this latter case, standards would be monitored through the 'leadership ladder' (Williams, personal communication). The major issue facing a British leadership is whether the aim of training is to improve services or to confront the moral issues which society presents to us (Kendrick 1989).

At the start of the 1990s, it is clear that normalisation training in Britain has reached something of a crossroads. The situation of a few years ago where a small number of pioneers carried out this work no longer applies. The large number of people now involved makes diversification inevitable. Radical new thinking is necessary if the positive elements of diversity are to be encouraged, without fragmenting the momentum for better services.

REFERENCES

Baldwin, S. (1985) 'Sheep in wolf's clothing: Impact of Normalisation teaching on human service providers', *International Journal of Rehabilitation and Research* 8, 2: 131–42.

Brown, H., and Alcoe, J. (1986) *New Lifestyles*: training packs for staff working with (i) People with Learning Difficulties, (ii) People with Mental Health Problems, (iii) Elderly People, Brighton: Pavilion Publishing Ltd.

Brown, H., with Bailey, R. and Brown, V. (1986–90) *Bringing People Back Home: a series of video assisted training programmes for staff in new services for People with Learning Difficulties*, Bexhill: SETRHA.

Burleigh, M. (1990) 'Nazi Euthanasia', *History Today*, Feb. 11–16.

Clifford, P. (1987) *Why I Haven't Joined the Normies*, The Bulletin of the South East Thames Psychiatric Rehabilitation Interest Group (S.P.R.I.N.G.), April.

Cocks, E. (1988) *Training and Evaluation for Change Group Project*, Evaluation Report, Perth.

Hoskins, S. (1989) *Outcomes*: a training game based on the Five Accomplishments, Bexhill: SETRHA.

Hudson, B. (1990) 'Better out than in?', *The Health Service Journal* 16 August: 1220–1.

Kendrick, M. (1989) *Personal Communication*, The Institute for Leadership and Community Development, Northampton MA, USA.

Klee, E. (1983) 'Euthanasie' im NS Staat die 'Vernichtung lebenswerten Lebens', Frankfurt.

Kristiansen, K. (1988) Dyffryn Gardens Introductory PASS Workshop, UK PASS, South Wales.

Kristiansen, K., and Tyne, A. (1985) 'Using PASS in Organisational Change', David Salomons House, unpublished.

Lemmer, W., and Braisby, D. (1990) 'Accomplishments for people in service transformation: An experiment in transitions training', *Health Services Journal*, November.

Lifton, R.J. (1986) *The N.A.Z.I. Doctors*, Papermac.

O'Brien, J. (1987) 'A guide to life style planning: Using the Activities Catalogue to integrate services and natural support systems', in B.W. Wilcox and G.T. Bellamy (eds) *The Activities Catalogue: An alternative curriculum for youth and adults with severe disabilities*, Baltimore: Brookes.

O'Brien, J., and Lyle, C. (1989) *Framework for Accomplishments*, Georgia, USA: Responsive Systems Associates.

O'Brien, J., and Tyne, A. (1981) *The Principle of Normalisation: A foundation for effective services*, London: Campaign for Mentally Handicapped People and Community and Mental Handicap Educational and Research Association.

O'Brien, J., and Wolfensberger, W. (1978) *CAPE: Standards for Citizen Advocacy Program Evaluation*, The Canadian Association for the Mentally Retarded.

Pilling, D. (1990) *Personal Communication*, Goldsmiths College, University of London.

Tyne, A. (1989) 'Normalisation: The next steps', *Community Living* 3: 7–8.

Wainwright, T. (1986) 'Normalisation – a valuable set of ideas', *SPRING* newsletter 6: 28–33.

Williams, P. (1990) *Personal Communication*, CMHERA.

Wolfensberger, W. (1972) *The Principle of Normalisation in Human Services*, Toronto: National Institute on Mental Retardation.

Wolfensberger, W. (1978) 'The ideal human service for a societally devalued group', *Rehabilitation Literature* 39, 1: 15–17.

Wolfensberger, W. (1980) 'The definition of Normalisation: Update, problems, disagreements and misunderstandings', in R.J. Flynn and K.E. Nitsch (eds) *Normalisation, Social Integration and Community Service*, Baltimore: University Park Press.

Wolfensberger, W. (1981) 'The extermination of handicapped people in World War II Germany', *Mental Retardation* 19, 1: 1–7.

Wolfensberger, W. (1983) 'Social Role Valorisation: A proposed new term for the principle of Normalisation', *Mental Retardation* 21, 6: 235–9.

Wolfensberger, W. (1984) 'A reconceptualisation of Normalisation as Social Role Valorisation', *Canadian Journal on Mental Retardation* 34, 7: 22–6.

Wolfensberger, W. (1985) 'Social Role Valorisation: A new insight, and a new term for Normalisation', *Australian Association for the Mentally Retarded Journal* 9, 1: 4–11.

Wolfensberger, W. (1987a) *The New Genocide of Handicapped and Afflicted People*, Syracuse University, New York: Training Institute for Human Service Planning and Change Agentry.

Wolfensberger, W. (1987b) 'How to Function with Personal Moral Coherency in a Disfunctional (Human Service) World', workshop offered by the Training Institute for Human Service Planning and Change Agentry, Syracuse University, New York.

Wolfensberger, W. (1990a) 'A most critical issue: Life or death', *Changes* 8, 1: 63–73.

Wolfensberger, W. (1990b) *TIPS:* Training Institute Publication Series, 9 April, Syracuse University, New York: Training Institute for Human Service Planning and Change Agentry.

Wolfensberger, W., and Glenn, L. (1973) *Program Analysis of Service Systems, a Method for the Quantitative Evaluation of Human Services*, 2nd Edition, Vol. I Handbook, Vol. II Field Manual, Toronto: National Institute on Mental Retardation.

Wolfensberger, W., and Glenn, L. (1975) *Program Analysis of Service Systems, a Method for the Quantitative Evaluation of Human Services*, 3rd Edition, Vol. I Handbook, Vol. II Field Manual, Toronto: National Institute on Mental Retardation 1975, reprinted 1978.

Wolfensberger, W., and Thomas, S. (1983) *PASSING (Program Analysis of Service Systems Implementation of Normalization Goals)*, Normalization Criteria and ratings manual (2nd Edition), Toronto: National Institute on Mental Retardation.

3 Normalisation
From theory to practice

Alan Tyne

IDEAS, COMMITMENT AND ACTION

Normalisation is an idea which has greatly influenced thinking about services to people with disabilities and its influence continues. This history will be a somewhat personal account, linking the development of the idea, the growth of a social movement around it and the many cross-currents of change which have influenced thinking and practice.

Paradoxically it seems sensible to begin in the middle of the story and then to sketch in some of the things which happened before and after. In the early 1980s, it was still necessary to look to America or Scandinavia for practical applications of normalisation in services for people with learning difficulties. A growing engagement with the ideas had led groups of people to believe in the possibility of people with substantial disabilities living in ordinary housing with such support as they needed. But as yet, in the United Kingdom, there were few examples from which to learn and no pictures or stories to help people share a vision of a different future for people with disabilities. However, by the end of the 1980s, there were many examples to draw on, any amount of film and photograph, stories and research accounts with which to document the impact of the ideas. In eight or ten years, we moved from first envisaging the possibilities, to them being recognised as practical daily accomplishments in at least some people's lives.

Ted and Alan (both men in their late fifties) had lived with elderly parents until, for a variety of reasons, they had to move into a small residential institution in 1985. Here the two men found themselves sharing a room and began to think together about moving back out into community life. Many meetings were held involving the two men and the people who knew them well. Since Alan has great difficulties with hearing and speech, it was important for people to take their time. Careful notes were kept on large posters so everyone concerned knew what was happening and could remember what had been said. It was felt that both men were beginning to lose many of the skills they once possessed and that they were missing the ordinary opportunities which a life in their local community had once brought them. A plan began to evolve for Ted and Alan to move into a flat which they would share.

A suitable flat was found with a friendly and helpful landlord. A solicitor drew up a proper rental agreement for the two men. Many different people were involved in the long process of getting the flat ready, getting furniture together and finally moving in. Both men enjoyed the quiet times in their new home and the photographs and memories of the busy days of planning and preparation. Part of their welfare benefits were used to pay two part-time helpers. One of these women has known the two men for a long time. She and her family are good friends to Alan and Ted. She usually helps with shopping, and her family, who live nearby, often make social calls to see the two men. The people in the Post Office have been particularly helpful in supporting Alan and Ted in managing their finances. A friend who has known Ted for many years calls regularly for a drink at their local pub. Alan has joined the congregation of a local church.

Life might have continued for a long time in this way if Ted had not had to go into hospital for several months for major heart treatment. Extra support was mobilised for Alan, who began to enjoy living on his own. When Ted returned, both men agreed they would be happier living apart. Some time later, they lived in separate flats, but within close proximity to each other. They are still friends and see each other regularly. They have had to make some compromises – each now gets less paid staff help than before, but each has new friends and contacts and new directions opening up in their lives. Ted and Alan continue to surprise us in their capacity to develop new skills and to meet new challenges.

In 1980, Susan lived in an institutional ward for 'violent females' – a place where the furniture was bolted to the floor and where every door was locked. Susan has no hearing and very little sight since her birth in 1940. She has virtually no communication skills, only a few signs. She does have a caring family who have stayed close by visiting her throughout her life, but her hospital records are a sad catalogue of emotional distress and much neglect. A chance came for her to move from the institution to a house with much support, including full-time staff. The transition was long and careful and Susan dictated the pace of change. In time, it was possible to meet her again, but now in the lounge of her new home where she entertained people to tea. An old dolls-pram, her only possession in the hospital, had been discarded in favour of a Hoover, dusters and polish.

Susan had discovered things she is good at, things in which she can make a contribution to the lives of others around her. She found a job, not a glamorous job, but her cleaning work in a restaurant brought her something she had never before enjoyed – an income. She held down several other jobs before deciding to stay with this one. She likes to spend her money on cosmetics and clothes. She has had to learn about many of the risks of everyday life – traffic and open fires for instance. The people who know her well have also had to learn what it means to take a 'reasonable risk'. Susan's disabilities have not diminished, in fact they may be growing more severe. She still has times of real emotional distress, but less often than she used to. She now has a room where she can go and be on her own and there is usually a friend or staff member who can sit with her to help bear her grief and unhappiness when it overwhelms her. The biggest difference is that it is now easy to meet and get to know Susan and this has led to many more people and opportunities in her life.

Neil works with five others in a small co-operative of woodworkers. They design and make unique decorative panels. In the workshop most of the daily interactions focus around the job in hand. There is little leisure time as it is a busy working place with orders to fulfil and a living to be made. They try to work as a co-operative of equals. This is not always easy when some people work a lot more quickly, consistently and productively than others. Neil has lived all his life in a caring family and more recently in a hostel which has a warm and accepting atmosphere.

Neil's life had taught him to wait while things were done for him and he met few situations which demanded anything of him. He had grown used to a living where his real poverty was masked by caring. In the co-operative he is a much loved and respected member and his kindness and humour make the day go well for everyone. He is skilled at drawing some of the designs for the panels. However, everyone is beginning to be aware that if he is to stay, then he has to learn to work hard, sustain his efforts and finish a job properly. Neil too is beginning to be aware of this. He is beginning to wonder if living in a flat would bring some of the same freedoms he has each day in the workshop. He is beginning to face the many personal decisions he will have to make and the commitments and responsibilities he will have to undertake. The 1990s will be a time of great change in his life but now Neil has many friends to help him with the exploration.

By the age of sixteen, John had lived in an impressive number of places, all of which had eventually rejected him and passed him to another. His records show that rarely a year passed without some new diagnosis being made, a greater variety and amount of drugs prescribed to control his behaviour and longer periods of time spent confined away from others or being physically restrained. His life had become a vicious circle in which every effort he made to control his own environment was met with more punishment, and in turn he responded with more anger against himself, against other people and against his surroundings. Experts were recommending he should either be locked away in a secure hospital with grown men, or very heavily sedated. Ominously, the latter recommendation added 'permanently if necessary'.

Nursing staff at one hospital who knew him well gathered together to try and rescue John from this crisis in his life. Five young male staff were recruited to share their lives with John by making a home together in a flat in the hospital grounds. At first John met only these people, no one else. For six months they patiently built trusting relationships with him. During the next two years this circle around him slowly began to grow. Others came to live in his house and some of the original group moved away, though not completely out of his life. He began to use classes at a local college, visit a community centre and through this began to meet other people including women, older people and young children, with whom he could build new relationships.

Time has passed and some of John's most important relationships are still the first few people who chose to live with him. He spends time at their homes and with their families and friends. He now lives in a small house near the hospital, which he shares with another young man. They have staff always with them. His circle of ties and connections with the community remains the same. The nursing staff say they have gone about as far as they can to rescue John from a fate which once seemed almost inevitable. Most people who know him well think that the pain and the hurt he felt through most of his childhood will mean that he will need continued help for many more years. Everyone is convinced that professional services cannot provide the major things which John needs in his life and it is now time for other people to begin to take responsibility. As yet, they are only just beginning to explore the alternative of building and supporting a community life around John in which he will have an integral and valued part.

These are not stories of perfection. Each is a story of struggle and endeavour towards something that remains elusive and at best unclear. Each involves major compromises that no-one really wanted. However, the stories are of major changes in the lives of some people with handicaps, changes which have increased their options and pointed the way to possible and desirable futures that could not previously have been imagined. In none of these stories was the major difference made by either cleverer technologies or by remarkable additional resources. Most of the difference was made by people coming to see and understand Ted and Alan, Susan, Neil and John differently. The vision for a new future became real as people took on a commitment to build new relationships in the lives of Ted, Alan and the others – and so things began to change.

Looking back over thirty years, not so much has changed (more of this shortly). What seems to have made the 1980s stand out was the growth and diffusion of a movement which encouraged this new vision of people and their possibilities, a preparedness among many individuals to engage directly and personally with the lives of people with substantial disabilities.

THE 1970s – PROLOGUE TO CHANGE

In the 1970s, public policy had responded to three kinds of pressures (Tyne 1982) – those generated by the scandals of abuse and neglect in the 1960s, the growing strength of the parent movement and the influence of developing professionalism in services. The immediate impact was seen in policies like 'Better Services for the Mentally Handicapped' (HMSO, Cmnd 4683) and the 1971 Education Act. These defined the situation of people with handicaps in terms of their need for professionally controlled facilities, such as beds, day-places; or in terms of services – assessment, therapy (of a thousand different kinds), treatment, supervision and training. There followed an explosion of interest in the situation of people with learning difficulties and many young professionals were drawn to work in a field which was beginning to claim public attention after years of denial and embarrassment. Cash followed the professionals and working with people with mental handicaps became an exciting prospect.

New people and new ideas early in the 1970s began to create their own crises. The medical profession had previously exerted a wide influence but now had less than a hundred consultants in the specialism and faced acute problems of training and recruitment (CMH 1978). Many were of the 'old school' of medical autocracy which was fiercely challenged by newer professional groups with increased confidence – nurses, teachers, social workers, instructors, psychologists and others. As these battles over medical control and the medical model began to be fought and won, so the professionals turned their attention to one another – how could such a disparate group of ambitious individuals, anxious to prove the worth of their particular discipline, learn to work together? Health and social service reorganisations and the growth of interest in joint planning and funding posed still greater challenges. Throughout the 1970s, professionals were absorbed with the intricacies and etiquette of multi-disciplinary working – subject of many conferences, study-days and learned papers. Reorganisation of professional work into community teams focused attention on team-work. A whole new specialism in 'team-building' emerged, demanding attendance at more courses, seminars and training days.

THE IMPACT OF TWENTY YEARS OF CHANGE

The developments of the 1970s undoubtedly effected changes in the lives of some people with handicaps, yet as we start the 1990s, many still remain in institutional environments for most of their days. The overall numbers in residential institutions have actually increased over the last twenty to thirty years, including the figures for local authority and private and voluntary provision. Many more people are likely to spend their daytimes in large mixed-purpose 'day-institutions'. The average size of residential institutions has declined somewhat, with many combinations of '24-bed' units. Some at least have developed areas where there is a markedly improved physical environment and there has been massive investment in the buildings which house people.

Yet the quality of these institutions has been largely unexamined. It is as if, having declared a policy of moving away from institutional care, policy makers have turned their attention away from measuring the quality of what happens within those institutions that remain. A superficial tour will quickly reveal, to the most casual observer, conditions of intolerable poverty, contrasting starkly with the growing affluence of many citizens during the 1980s.

One of the most systematic ways in which these environments have been documented during the 1980s has been through their use as 'practice placements' for participants in PASS and PASSING training workshops (see Lindley and Wainwright, this volume). The results of around 200 of these practice assessments have been analysed (Williams 1988) and they present an alarming picture of life in large congregate settings with minimal dignity, few activities which would contribute to development and growth and little contact with the outside world. The attempt to upgrade these institutions has paid a great deal of attention to what goes in (money, equipment, qualifications and even good intentions) but very little to what effect this has on the lives of the people they serve.

The agendas of the 1970s focused on the development of the professions and limited reform of the institutions. These agendas continued throughout the 1980s as the major preoccupation of policy makers and planners. Added to them though is a new rhetoric of 'Community Care', and some new possibilities for service managers to shift resources in new directions. A careful accounting of what resources have indeed been shifted and of who has benefited from these changes has yet to be done. Few institutions have actually closed and for some, closure has been achieved largely by transferring clients to other institutions (CMH 1986).

Since the 1970s, there has been little systematic documentation of the real changes in the lives of people who rely on services. What can be said is that whether living in institutions or remaining in the family home, most people still find it difficult to get specialised and expert help if they have a major problem with communication, getting about, learning complex skills or dealing with relationships and emotions. Few have any real options about where to live or who to live with, or about what job to do. Families worrying about the future of their disabled son or daughter are still, in the 1990s, faced with a similar range of more-or-less unsatisfactory compromises as would have faced them in the 1960s.

The stories of Alan, Ted, Susan, Neil and John have been influenced by the principle of normalisation. Not only are their stories very different from one another and falling short of ideals in many ways, but they are also not yet typical. Whilst some research (Felce and Toogood 1988; Flynn 1989) has begun to describe the quality of small projects supporting people with handicaps in community living, we know little yet about how many people are being so supported. The stories recounted here could probably only be told of a relatively small number of people.

THE EFFECT OF NEW WAYS OF THINKING

Normalisation as an idea to be learned, discussed, worked with, came late in the 1970s. Historically, it was a critical moment when many things came together to create the right climate for the ideas. There was a power vacuum in services, with medical consultants in decline and the new professions still testing their horns against one another. There was also an ideological vacuum, with many people doubting the new dogmas of community teams and community units developed by the National Development Group and the Development Team. There was a policy vacuum, as reviews of progress since 'Better Services' revealed major shortfalls and a loss of impetus. On the positive side, EXODUS (the campaign to get children out of long-stay hospitals), the 'An Ordinary Life' group at the King's Fund Centre and the Jay Committee were meeting and disseminating new ideas and the example of ENCOR in the USA was creating a buzz of excitement.

We can now see that the effect of these new ways of thinking, if measured in terms of the numbers of people whose lives have been changed, or the redirection of major aspects of social policy, has not been great. Indeed, as described elsewhere (Whitehead, this volume) these things have continued to be affected mainly by other political and social influences. But the effect of normalisation can be seen in the individual lives of Alan and Ted, Susan, Neil and John. In each of these stories, normalisation significantly influenced people's thinking and working practices.

First, it created a decided focus on the life situation of people with handicaps. Disciplines like PASS and PASSING (and others derived from them) required people to 'take off their professional hats' for a while, and to spend time with handicapped people trying to gain an understanding of how life really was for them. They required people to face up to the realities of life for handicapped people, in contrast to the often over-optimistic schemes and dreams of the professionals.

Second, it offered a framework for asking questions and for problem solving. Normalisation does not offer ready answers, but it does set questions. As the deceptively simple idea that you should 'seek valued ends through the use of valued means' was explored, it led to extensive questioning of professional and service practices. As normalisation was elaborated, many conflicts and inconsistencies were revealed, so that problem-solving within the framework of normalisation has seldom been a simple or quick business, but has required struggle and effort. As people have accepted the challenges and worked with them, so understandings of the practical implications of normalisation have grown. It has been an evolving idea, not a fixed dogma, and sometimes the evolution has been painful and difficult.

Third, it began to create agendas for action – the movement towards the use of ordinary housing and community living, the push towards real work and employment and a new focus on the importance of relationships. Other agendas connected with the normalisation movement, notably citizen advocacy and self-advocacy, started to develop and included in these changes came a re-evaluation of the nature of community.

Fourth, it created networks of people – in truth, a social movement of a unique kind. A leadership developed that stretched across and beyond service boundaries. Normalisation was not the possession of any particular profession or discipline. It gave a basis for understanding problems and participating in decision making that did not rely on professional credentials. Everyone could share the vision of a new future for people – people with disabilities, parents and friends, interested citizens, service workers, managers and planners, policy makers. It has evolved largely through people directly engaged in trying to make the ideas work in practice and in their own lives.

NORMALISATION AND POLICY DEVELOPMENT

At another level, the idea of normalisation has had a very different kind of impact. Initially, academics and professionals took a somewhat aloof and distant interest. The ideas began to be disseminated in the United Kingdom by a tiny organisation, Community and Mental Handicap Educational and Research Association (CMHERA) – surviving on short-term grants and borrowed office space. But the strength of the organisation lay in its networks, not in its name or its premises. Its workshops (see Lindley and

Wainwright, this volume) proved to be an effective training ground, not just for the participants who turned up to learn about normalisation, but also for those who were group leaders, and who in turn took over the leadership of future events.

As the ideas became established in this country, so people took a more critical interest. Doctors, and some policy analysts (Malin 1987), dubbed them as 'left wing' – seeking to overturn established social patterns and hierarchies. Others (see Smith and Brown 1989) seemed to be accusing it of the opposite – obliging handicapped people to fit the norms and expectations of a greedy and unjust society. People with strong religious views said it was too secular and failed to recognise the unique value and worth of each individual, regardless of their social roles. A similar critique regarding the failure to recognise individuality came from radical voices in the independent living movement of disabled people. At workshops, secular workers criticised its values-based approach as 'quasi-religious'. Professionals of a variety of affiliations said it was anti-nurse, anti-social work, anti-medical and anti-professional. Normalisation became the basis for intense and varied debate.

It is not accidental of course that this debate about values should coincide with the first decade of Thatcherite government policies. It was a time when values of all kinds were up for question and debate. The opportune entry of normalisation into the social policy agenda in the late 1970s meant that it came to be the arena in which the debate about service values was staged. As a nation, however, we are probably still ill-prepared for a debate about values. Half a century ago, R.H. Tawney (1922) pointed to our national preoccupation with practical things and our suspicion of 'theory' in any form. One of the effects of talking so explicitly about values was that many people felt themselves 'upstaged'. It was as if, in pointing to the values underlying service organisations' behaviour, they were being accused of immorality or having no existing values. To others, brought up in the climate of 'public service' in the post-war welfare state, with its careful separation of Church and state, the whole 'values' debate seemed like a dangerous return to the muddled and selective do-gooding of the past.

The professions responded in different ways. For many, normalisation provided a programme for thought and action which seemed helpful in responding to the challenges of change in the 1980s. The academic and professional critiques of normalisation did not stop practitioners from signing up in numbers for courses and workshops. There have been continuous efforts to maintain the quality of the training events, against equally continuous pressures to make them cheaper, more accessible, less reliant on skilled leadership and less demanding of participants. The paradox is that the workshops, which were safeguarded by CMHERA and its supporters to be a fierce independent challenge to the official service system, are at risk of being colonised and taken over by that same system. Increasingly, professionals come to regard their PASS/PASSING experience as a credential, something to be included in their curriculum vitae when applying for the next job.

Probably more dangerous has been the somewhat hasty adoption of normalisation as a new 'technical fix'. When normalisation is adopted as if it were a technology or professional tool, particular elements of the ideas are sometimes taken and extended to bizarre lengths. So people who it is reasonable to assume will always need substantial amounts of help in their daily lives are subjected to lengthy 'independence-training' as a precondition to community living – a process where they often experience repeated failure. Others are denied special help which they need, on the grounds that it 'wouldn't be normal'. Others still experience a great deal of boredom, frustration and inactivity in community settings because this is said to be 'encouraging choice'. Some wait interminably whilst professionals argue about the 'right grouping', the 'right size' and other particularities. Others are placed into houses in which enormous attention is given to the setting and environment, but almost none at all to relationships and community membership, which may be seen as 'not our job'.

There are also dangers in the wholesale adoption of normalisation. Few professions are now without the obligatory potted version of normalisation somewhere in their basic training syllabus. Managers and planners jump to the quick conclusion that normalisation must mean community care and there is seldom a post advertised in services for people with learning difficulties that does not claim adherence to normalisation. Authorities, pressed to develop community services quickly, have little time to invest in new learning and may send one member of staff on a normalisation course to act as a messenger. In an age of short-term, quick-fix thinking, there is little incentive to think seriously about the scale and the long-term nature of the changes which normalisation proposes. New services are launched optimistically with staff who have gleaned something of the challenge which normalisation sets out, but with an inadequate understanding of the conflicts and compromises that await them and little grounding in ideas, which would help them tackle those challenges. Many community services are now beginning to run into the inevitable disappointments, with little to see them through. There is a very real risk of an equally headlong rush back into institutional provision, as a response to this failure.

In the main, these distortions come about when people erect a barrier, put a professional distance between themselves and the people whom they serve. By doing that, they become capable of using normalisation as if it were a professional technology for effecting changes in other people's lives, without themselves getting involved. Something in their professional training and detachment gets in the way of individuals understanding the effects of their actions in others' lives. The danger is that we may develop all the traditional arrogance of professionals – 'we know best; we're trained so we "know" and don't have to go on learning; we can effect changes in people's lives without getting involved with the whole person'.

Over the next few years the movement faces considerable challenges. We need to recognise some of the things we have not done well. In our teaching, for instance, have we been better at telling people what *not* to do rather than help them use disciplines creatively to invent new patterns of community life? The challenge for the small group of people who continue to present the PASS/PASSING training as a focus for teaching normalisation will be how to maintain its freshness and independence and to make it accessible to everyone, including people with disabilities, their families and friends and to ordinary concerned citizens.

'Learning by doing' about community living suggests a whole new way of thinking about services. History has taught communities to look to professional services to care for people with disabilities; twenty years of working for change has taught us that services by themselves can never be enough. We need to invent new ways of working with communities which build and support community competence rather than undermine it. In doing that, our competence as community members may be of more help to us than our 'professional' qualifications. Detached and self-preoccupied professionalism will only get in the way.

We will also need to bear in mind that despite years, centuries even, of determined struggle by articulate but disempowered groups, we still live in a society with a power structure which largely continues to discriminate against women, black and poor people. And this is the society we are asking to be more welcoming to elders and people with disabilities! If we engage with the struggle for change which is central to the principle of normalisation, we will need to face the meanness, unfairness, untidiness and fickleness of community life in the faith that we may change some of it, some of the time, for some people. Mostly that is going to mean each of us making long-term commitments to the bit of community life that is close to us.

Critiques of normalisation do not seem to have seriously impeded the growth of a movement that has linked the people who struggled to create stories such as those described at the beginning of this chapter. Probably this is because the critiques have happened at some remove from the lives of people with disabilities. There is a certain rarefied detachment about some of the debate which has not made much sense to Alan and Ted and the others, and to the people closely engaged in their lives. The power of the normalisation idea and of the movement which has grown around it has lain not just in its capacity for problem solving and analysis, but in the invitation it offers to people and communities to engage their lives directly with those of people with disabilities; people who are at risk of being rejected, marginalised, excluded, oppressed. The ideas have become the basis for personal and collective behaviour which has helped create the stories told here. The impact of the ideas on the policy system is much harder to detect. The main difference between now and 1960 is that then, perhaps there was an excuse for the way things were. Now there is none – and the stories of Alan and Ted, Susan, Neil and John stand as testimony to the way things could be.

REFERENCES

CMH (1978) 'Who's Consulted?', Enquiry Paper No. 8., London: Values into Action.
CMH (1986) Alison Wertheimer, 'Hospital closures in the eighties', London: VIA.
Felce, D., and Toogood, S. (1988) 'Close to Home', BIMH Publications.
Flynn, M.C. (1989) *Independent Living for Adults with Mental Handicap: A place of my own*, London: Cassell Educational.
Malin, N. (1987) 'Principles, Policy and Practice', in N. Malin (ed.) *Reassessing Community Care*, Beckenham: Croom Helm.
Smith, H., and Brown, H. (1989) 'Whose community. Whose care?', in A. Brechin and J. Walmsley (eds) *Making Connections: Reflecting on the lives and experiences of people with learning difficulties*, The Open University, Hodder and Stoughton Educational.
Tawney, R.H. (1922) *The Acquisitive Society*, London: G. Bell and Sons.
Tyne, A. (1982) 'Community care and mentally handicapped people', in A. Walker (ed.) *Community Care – The Family, the State and Social Policy*, Blackwell and Robertson.
Williams, P. (1988) Unpublished paper. CMHERA, 69, Wallingford Road, Goring, Oxon.

4 The social origins of normalisation

Simon Whitehead

Ideas, beliefs or concepts do not appear from nowhere. Although they may develop around specific issues their origins lie within a complex web of personal, social and political variables. This chapter seeks to explain why it was that normalisation became an influential concept in the development of human services. Normalisation did not arise in isolation, but was the distillation of significant ideas, movements and attitudes that came to the fore in the post-war period. It arose partly out of international concerns, reflected in the human and civil rights movements and the new sociology of the 1960s and also as a result of social and political changes specific to the United Kingdom (although these have their clear parallels in other Western countries where the concept became a force for change). These background issues need to be traced and the connections between them defined, in order to understand the limitations imposed on normalisation by its historical origins.

A historical overview is necessary both to unravel the significant perspectives which contributed to its development and to understand the complementary agendas which led to its becoming an influential and lasting movement for change.

RIGHTS – A KEY CONCEPT

Human rights have long been the subject of philosophical discussion and dissertations and they are enshrined in different forms in constitutions and legal systems; however their significance in understanding the origins of normalisation only emerged after the Second World War. There is a general consensus that the deprivations of the Depression in the 1930s, and the atrocities committed by Hitler's regime, led both to political changes and a determination that rights of minority groups across the world should be protected in the future. This was enshrined in the Articles that make up the Charter of the United Nations (1948), and more specifically in the United

Nations Declaration of Human Rights adopted in 1948. Although these documents did not in themselves have legal status, they led to the enactment of human rights treaties, such as the Covenant on Civil and Political Rights (1966) and the International Covenant on Economic, Social and Cultural Rights (1966) which contain some fundamental statements that are binding in Great Britain under international law. Similarly, the European Convention on Human Rights (1950) has been used by the European Court of Human Rights to make decisions which have changed laws and practice in this country. In 1971, the United Nations adopted the Declaration on the Rights of Mentally Retarded Persons (1971), recognising that the earlier declarations were not specific enough to protect this group of people.

The issue of human rights erupted in the United States after the Second World War as the civil rights movement became an undeniable force for change. The prominent role played by black soldiers in the United States army highlighted the inequalities for them when they returned home and by 1948, President Truman was campaigning on their behalf. By the mid-1950s the battle over equality and segregation was being fought in the courts and when Southern states resisted the changes and found loopholes in court decisions, the battle moved to the streets – of Dallas, Watts, Detroit and other places. At the heart of this conflict was the massive contradiction of the American dream – on the one hand its emphasis on equality and human rights and on the other the grim reality for many, especially black people whose lives were characterised by poverty and inequality in virtually all spheres of life, exacerbated by dependence on crime and drugs.

The black civil rights movement provided a model for other disadvantaged groups in the United States and elsewhere. Many young men returned from the Second World War with physical disabilities, forerunners of the articulate veterans of Korea and Vietnam. Improved medical techniques had kept them alive and improved technology enabled them to return to society. The major polio epidemics of the early 1950s further raised the profile of people with disabilities and highlighted their lack of rights. But changes were hindered by the rapid growth of professionalised and specialist services which depicted people as medical problems to be treated and rehabilitated. Whilst many concerned parents, friends and others formed organisations to campaign on behalf of people with particular disabilities, few disabled people were directly involved. Thus although a notion of rights was recognised in the abstract, disability services remained located within a disempowering, paternalistic framework.

Nonetheless, young people with disabilities made it clear that they wanted to resume a normal community life and recognised that this would only happen if they fought collectively to regain control over their own lives. In tracing the development of Disabled Peoples' International (DPI)

– an organisation formed in 1981 to create a united voice for disabled people – Driedger (1989) points to the important influence of four international organisations of disabled people formed in the early 1950s: the World Federation of the Deaf, the International Federation of the Blind, People First International and the Fédération Internationale des Mutilés, des Invalides du Travail and des Invalides Civil. Throughout the 1960s and 1970s these organisations influenced both the international movement for civil rights for people with disabilities and the development of both national and local organisations. In Britain, this culminated in the formation of the British Council of Organisations of Disabled People in 1981.

These organisations, like those which emerged involving black people, women, tenants of rented accommodation and a number of other oppressed minority groups, were fighting both for the basic human rights enjoyed by other people and for a fundamental change in attitudes. They wanted a move away from the patronage and pitying accorded to them within professionalised services and by the public at large, both of which divested them of power over their own lives.

CHALLENGING ACADEMIC CONSERVATISM

The challenge to the conservative attitudes of the 1950s was also reflected in the study of sociology, particularly in the United States. Until then the dominant force in sociology had been the structural-functionalist school, epitomised by the work of Talcott Parsons (1951). After the Second World War a consensus had emerged about reconstruction and working together to rebuild society which fed into this conservative and paternalistic theory, assuming that all the various functions and institutions of a society worked together as part of a cohesive whole: if something existed, then it must serve a function that helped maintain and preserve society. Thus such issues as criminality, mental illness or other disabilities were seen as pieces of a jigsaw – static and uncontentious conditions, which fitted into the overall picture of society as a cohesive entity.

In the 1960s a major challenge to the structural-functionalists emerged. This rejected the inherent conservatism of the approach and concentrated on social processes, rather than institutions and functions. Labelling theory, characterised by the work of Goffman (1961), looked at these categories in terms of how and why people were defined by others and explored the effect of this labelling process on people's subsequent behaviour. Labelling essentially creates deviance or abnormality because the individual adjusts his or her behaviour to that ascribed to them by the label. Others react to the individual on the basis of their label, which in turn exacerbates the deviant behaviour and is communicated to a wider audience – and the deviancy is 'amplified'. Thus developed the concept of the vicious circle, or self-fulfilling prophecy in relation to social behaviour which was to greatly influence Wolfensberger in his development of normalisation.

Deviancy theory, taken up by sociologists such as Becker (1964), Lemert (1967) and Cohen (1971), broadened the concept of labelling theory to any group which deviated from the 'norm' and these views began to challenge traditional institutional and professional approaches to people previously described as medical or social problems. They relocated the problem in the processes of institutional or professional definition – in other words the problem is created by those seeking to do something about it. Deviancy theory owed much to two other sociological schools of thought that were in themselves major challenges to the functional approaches; one was symbolic interactionism which grew out of the work of Meade (1934). This focused on the crucial part played by the symbolic understanding of how others perceive you ('me') in determining the true nature of self ('I'). Second, ethnomethodology (see for example Garfinkel (1967)) sought to understand the actions of individuals in the context of the meaning attached to every-day events in their lives.

These ideas led to changes in thinking in a number of areas of social policy. They connected and gave credence to the wider social movements which sought to challenge traditional values and approaches to life and its difficulties. It led to radical new views of psychiatry (characterised by the work of R.D. Laing (1964), Szasz (1962) and epitomised by Kesey's novel *One Flew Over the Cuckoo's Nest* (1962)). Studies of criminology were radicalised by the work of Cohen and Taylor (1972), amongst others, and traditional social work focusing on individual pathology gave way to the development of community work as a viable alternative.

Thus in the 1950s and 1960s the civil rights movements, together with the new theories in sociology, combined to produce change on an international level. These changes included the sense that all human beings should be seen as individuals in their own right and this prompted a sense of injustice about some of the customs, practices and attitudes which were prevalent. Society responded to the exciting new explanations of why some people behaved the way they did, or were the way they were. In relation to the development of normalisation, however, these changes are still only part of the picture and there are a number of other contextual matters to consider.

THE GENERAL SOCIAL CONTEXT

In the post-war period there were two strong social movements which, irrespective of party politics, were strongly to influence public attitudes and opinion: the idea of all human beings being individual in their own right, worthy of the same dignity and respect as others; and the notion of welfare that recognised that some people's needs were greater than others, and that the state had a role in providing or ensuring that appropriate supports were available to enable people to live as ordinary human beings.

The Depression of the 1930s, with both its economic and social consequences, had shocked people in the United Kingdom. The social injustice of the situations in which so many found themselves was unacceptable to most people regardless of political or social persuasion. The deprivation of the Depression was then followed by the horror of a world war, which had two galvanising effects. The first was to highlight the extremes of depravity and inhumanity to which other humans could sink, in the atrocities perpetrated by Hitler's regime, and the Japanese in the East; and secondly, to illustrate the achievements that could be made through collective action – working together to support each other in the defeat of a common enemy.

However, the promise of radical change in the late 1940s gradually evaporated in the 1950s. The generation who had fought the war recognised the need for some safeguards, but as affluence gradually returned, the will to rethink existing and traditional values and structures diminished. It was essentially the next generation who reacted to both the horrors of war and oppression, and the complicity of their parents in maintaining social institutions and systems which operated with many of the hallmarks of repressive, discriminatory attitudes. Europe saw the most extreme reaction in a new generation who resorted to violence against the state – the Red Army Faction, the Baader–Meinhof Gang. But reaction reverberated throughout Britain as well, and no traditional institutions were spared: it was seen publicly in the emergence of anti-establishment youth culture in the 1950s and 1960s, and the development of the so-called permissive society, with its liberal values of peace and love. It was seen in social studies of institutions, such as *Pentonville* by the Morrises (1963), and *Sans Everything* by Barbara Robb (1967), which connected new sociological thinking with real social concerns. In all walks of life there was rebellion and ferment, as anyone who attended traditional British Public Schools or Universities in the late 1950s and 1960s will testify.

THE POLITICAL CONTEXT

The crucial development of the Welfare State spanned these two periods of radical thought. Bruce (1987) described the Welfare State as being

> the sum of efforts over many years to remedy the practical social difficulties and evils of a modern system of economic organisation which grew with but little regard for the majority of those who became

involved in it . . . . It is organised to ensure the well-being of its citizens and to use their resources to that end.

(Bruce 1961: 17)

It is possible to understand, in the immediate aftermath of the Second World War, why there was support for the Beveridge Plan of 1942 and a mandate for the Labour Government to enact, in 1945, the universalist Beveridge principles into the National Assistance Act, and bring about the birth of the National Health Service. For the first time, a firm link was made between the social and the economic in the politics of social welfare.

However, as Britain passed through the austerity of reconstruction following the war, and met the renewed impact of the cost of armaments and the effect of inflation during the early 1950s, the limitations imposed by finite public expenditure led to a back-lash against the universalist policies inherent in the Beveridge proposals. Ironically, as affluence increased, the universalist notion of the welfare state became increasingly threatened. Even in an affluent society, the cost and complexity of running a global welfare system seemed overwhelming. So whilst politically there remained some humanity and enlightenment – characterised for example by improved child care legislation, the 1959 Mental Health Act and Enoch Powell's 1961 speech about running down and replacing outdated long-stay Victorian asylums – the motivation and extent of the changes were brought under the control of economic factors. These in turn had their roots in political views about the extent of state intervention – a conflict between collectivist and market-based, *laissez-faire*, ideologies. By the late 1960s most politicians were agreed that wholly universal welfare benefits and services were unattainable, so selectivity and means testing were accepted. The ensuing arguments centred on the means of determining the selection, the extent of it, and the means of funding and providing what was deemed necessary.

By the 1970s, there appeared to be agreement that all was far from well with the welfare state. To the collectivists and Fabians it seemed that the state centralisation had concentrated too much power in essentially conservative institutions and professions, which, despite their benevolent intentions, were largely about social control. To the New Right, as it emerged, the certainties of state paternalism were questioned; as Clarke *et al.* (1987) have commented, the poor experienced this as oppressive, the well-off as expensive and wasteful. The concepts of unified social services, decentralisation and the idea of community care seemed to be accepted by all, although these contain essentially different political analyses, which were not well articulated or formulated. So politically, the 1970s left a political vacuum, or at least uncertainty about both the direction of welfare, and the mechanisms by which results could be achieved. There was little attempt to articulate what kind of outcomes were desirable for the recipients of social welfare services or for what political reasons they should be pursued.

THE COMMUNITY CARE CONTEXT

Thus the social policy objective of community care (as opposed to care in institutional settings) emerged in the United Kingdom without any clear sociological or political analysis. Early development took place in the field of mental handicap and less so in mental health services, where change has been slower. The history of services to people with learning difficulties illustrates the gradual refinement of the idea and indicates when normalisation became a relevant concept.

Prior to the nineteenth century, there was very little by way of provision of services for people with learning difficulties; although perceptions of and understanding about why some people seemed to develop more slowly than others will have varied, it can only be assumed that most lived in their family homes, or at least within local communities. Special and segregated provision did not develop until the Industrial Revolution which increased social mobility, smaller households and poverty in rapidly expanding urban areas. The emergence of groups unable, within the prevailing social systems, to work or contribute financially became more and more apparent. As many poor families struggled, the need for alternative provision for those seen as idiots and imbeciles became more pressing. At first, the response of early reformers was well-intentioned, and fashioned on the basis of an educational model; small asylums grew up with the objective of improving their residents, so that they might return to their communities. However, the promise of these early educationally orientated services was not fulfilled – it seemed they had misunderstood and underestimated the environmental factors which had led to people being unable to survive in the first place and the asylums and schools gradually became repressive and increasingly custodial institutions.

By the early part of this century, increasing numbers of people were unable to cope, unsupported, within the community which fuelled dangerous eugenic ideologies about increasing degeneracy and hereditary disabilities. Thus grew up the legacy that is still with us today, of large segregated institutions which, having begun as workhouses, changed with succeeding theories and models, to become asylums and ultimately 'subnormality' hospitals. Views about the cause and nature of learning disabilities changed from one in which the 'imbeciles' needed improvement, through to being the degenerate result of the sins of the parents or a reversion through a genetic fault to some subhuman species, to more recent location within a medical model: but the essential service response remained the same. People with learning difficulties who, for whatever reasons, were unable to remain with their families ended up in large segregated institutions, albeit with slightly differing interpretations over the years about why they were there.

It is only in the last forty years that this pattern of service provision and response has changed significantly. Although limited forms of community care developed in the first half of the twentieth century (e.g. people literally being 'farmed out'), it was not until the 1950s and 1960s that the concept really developed. The Royal Commission on Mental Illness and Mental Deficiency of 1954–7 (1957) actually used the term 'community care' to head one of the chapters of its report, that spelt out the local authority's duties in relation to the National Assistance Act, and the National Health Service Act. These duties were singled out as the Royal Commission considered in some detail the problems arising from the continued use of the large and often very old hospitals where many people lived. This emphasis on the inappropriateness of outdated long-stay hospitals was further articulated in a surprising and forceful speech by Enoch Powell in 1961, which was followed by the Community Care Blue Book in 1963. Although there was some scepticism about the real motives behind the desire to 'run down the old mental hospital' (i.e. cost saving), there was a shared view that the Victorian asylums really were no place for fellow human beings to live.

Through the 1960s, with social values changing dramatically, particularly amongst the young, and as the deviancy sociologists picked up from the work of Goffman (1961) the depersonalising and inhumane effects of large institutions, there was strong public condemnation of the abuses in hospitals which emerged at South Ockendon, Ely, Farleigh and Whittingham, and were publicly reported in the late 1960s. These gave renewed impetus towards community care, and in 1971 the government published 'Better Services for the Mentally Handicapped' (1971) which set clear targets for the development of alternative residential and day services.

At this stage, as Bayley pointed out in 1973, the alternatives to hospital were still largely conceptualised as state-run, segregated services, in the form of hostels and day centres. Little thought had been given to the meaning of 'community care', and little attention paid to the notions of integration into ordinary settings, relationships with families and friends, or the idea of employment and an 'ordinary life' for people with learning difficulties. The early 1970s saw an initial and rapid expansion in local authority services, followed by an equally rapid retrenchment as the economic situation deteriorated and the International Monetary Fund stepped in. This resulted in a slowing down of the development of the rather conservative alternative services, and a re-examination of priorities within local services which also coincided with an increasing cynicism about the apparent failure of the large public agencies to respond to the needs of individuals. Departments and agencies had become obsessed with systems approaches to service development, addressing problems by large-scale reorganisations, which paid scant regard to the impact of their services on the lives of people, or the wishes of those seeking help.

THE EMERGENCE OF NORMALISATION AS A FORCE FOR CHANGE

The time had not been ripe for normalisation until this point, because the understanding of learning disability had not gone beyond seeing it as an affliction which required treating, or an evil to be split off – explanations which avoided any notions of equal human rights, or examination of the social context which handicapped individuals with learning difficulties. It was the coming together of these different but connected contextual factors which provided the circumstances within which the concept of normalisation could emerge.

Thus it was appropriate and relevant that the concept of normalisation should appear in Britain in the mid-1970s, when there had developed a clear need for an ideological framework which:

(1) was clearly based on basic human values;
(2) took account of the social context in which people lived, in terms of its meaning and consequences for them;
(3) concentrated on the impact of services on the lives of the people they were designed to serve;
(4) challenged the traditional and paternalistic responses which characterised statutory services, and the professionals who ran them.

There is no doubt that the principle of normalisation has been of major significance as a force for change in human services throughout the 1980s, and remains so now. The test ultimately for any ideology which has been adopted at a particular point in time, and within a particular conflation of circumstances, is whether it is dynamic enough to learn from changing events, attitudes and situations, and adjust the content of both theory and practice accordingly.

Normalisation emerged as an influential concept in the field of learning difficulties in Britain during the late 1970s, its influence spreading rapidly through the early 1980s. Community care had, by then, become a specific and widely discussed policy objective, with the issuing of a significant Government Circular in 1983 (1983), following an earlier Green Paper (1981). Although the policy explicitly referred to the goal of running down the large hospitals, and to providing better quality community services, the political motivation was linked to the high costs of running traditional hospital services, the huge capital value of some of the old hospital sites, and a return to a *laissez-faire* market ideology which anticipated an alternative way to procure, provide and deliver services using the private sector. This was first articulated in the social welfare field in a speech made at Buxton in 1985 by the then Secretary of State for Health and Social Security, Norman Fowler.

However, whilst there were stringent reductions in public expenditure for economic and political reasons that posed a threat to the development of services, the free market individualism inherent in the New Right's approach found some common ground with service providers and planners. The desire to shed the yoke of paternalism, the emphasis on the needs of the individual, and giving people freedom of choice became common goals that bridged an otherwise huge political divide.

This provided the window of opportunity for those involved in developing services, for people with learning difficulties, based on an 'ordinary life' philosophy. It also enabled the principle of normalisation to be used in relation to other client/patient groups. There was some deep-rooted scepticism about the long-term political and economic motives of the Conservative government led by Mrs Thatcher based partly on a mistrust of the ultimate aim of a privatised service sector. There was also cynicism about the moral authoritarianism of the centre which would ultimately determine the extent and nature of 'self-help'. However, in the shorter term, there was consensus about some of the worst aspects of traditional services, and the importance of returning to an individualised needs-led approach.

Nor was there an effective political alternative in the early 1980s. Some Socialists recognised that the state, whilst providing welfare services, also kept people in a dependent and powerless state by doing so (a view echoed by the rapidly emerging women's and other self-help movements). Others were unclear how to develop *collectivist* policies that provided *individuals* with better support and services (see Dalley, this volume).

Wolfensberger's thesis on normalisation (1972), and the subsequent PASS (1975) and PASSING (1983) instruments, were the prime movers of change, but although they are still used today, and still have their place, the influence of normalisation cannot be ascribed to them alone and its continued ability to inspire high quality services depends on whether it will be possible to adjust and develop it. There is no doubt that as the idea of normalisation has spread and been adopted by so many people in service agencies and training curricula, it has slowly been diluted by the process of dissemination. This is both inevitable and regrettable as it can weaken its original message. However, it does also mean it is subjected to repeated analysis, scrutiny and evaluation; its limitations recognised; and its weaknesses addressed. This does not always please the purists, who may see innovations as an aberration; but there are inherent weaknesses emerging in the principle as time and events proceed.

Because normalisation is so closely allied to the deviancy school of sociology, it has tended to recreate the same difficulties in its relying on 'processes' to the exclusion of culture-specific considerations. Interactionists give little or no credence to the historical or social context in which events or behaviours occur and do not acknowledge that as these contexts change, these will themselves affect events and behaviour. Normative values (which are a 'given' in normalisation and deviancy theory) need to and do change; theories which assume such norms are defined, accepted and appropriate, are inherently conservative, and cannot explain or support variation or change.

Moreover, normalisation inadvertently maintains people as victims, implying that we should believe there will always be devalued victims (as defined by deviancy theories) – it would not need to exist as a principle otherwise. Thus there is a vested interest in believing there will always be people in a devalued state who by definition cannot get themselves out of it. This is characterised by the adoption of normalisation largely by professionals and service providers, rather than disabled people themselves. So, whilst services have moved away from a treatment model, they have only moved to an advocacy model – others speaking up on behalf of disabled people. There has not been a real shift in the balance of power as a direct result of normalisation. Although many of the values of the groups of disabled people who have organised themselves and sought changes in the way society treats them are the same as those of normalisation, normalisation itself has not contributed a great deal to the politics of empowerment.

Whilst the original exponents of normalisation in Scandinavia put great emphasis on individuality and choice, Wolfensberger's more sociologically conservative orientated theories put the specific impact of services on the lives of particular individuals as secondary to the wider social implications of devalued status. The individualism of the 1980s has led to more importance being attached to the impact of services on the lives of individuals, and positive value attached to the concept of choice. This problem has been addressed in the Framework for Accomplishment devised by John O'Brien (1987), which reinstates the impact of service systems on individuals as central, together with the importance of informed individual choice. There remains a tension around choices which relate to cultural values or norms which are not regarded as valued in the wider society or could be seen to be damaging to the person or others. The implication within normalisation that to redress the devalued status of people with learning difficulties, they should be encouraged to assume the cultural values of the majority whose roles and status are most valued, imposes its own limitations. This has become particularly apparent when normalisation has been applied to people from different ethnic backgrounds or to larger oppressed groups such as women. Then the theory has no room for the kind of cultural diversity and choice which many individuals wish to exercise in living their lives in different ways to those implicit in the dominant culture.

THE FUTURE

This chapter has sought to understand the historical and social policy context from which normalisation emerged, in order to understand why it developed and became influential at the time it did. Whilst drawing on the international context, the particular social and political circumstances in Britain were used to illustrate how normalisation became a significant force for change in the mid to late 1970s.

That influence has remained through the 1980s, and continues today. The work of John O'Brien more recently has enabled services to adopt the essential values and strengths of normalisation by being opportunistic within a dominant context of political individualism. There are, however, some key issues arising in the areas of, first, the empowerment of oppressed groups themselves through consciousness-raising, self-help, and political action, and, second, the definitions of community integration and community participation in a multi-racial, multi-cultural society – which suggest that the influence of normalisation may be overtaken unless it is redefined in the context of a new set of circumstances and social priorities.

REFERENCES

Bayley, M.J. (1973) *Mental Handicap and Community Care*, London: Routledge and Kegan Paul.

Becker, H. (1964) *The Other Side: Perspectives on deviance*, New York: The Free Press.

Better Services for the Mentally Handicapped (1971), Cmnd. 4683, London: HMSO.

Bruce, M. (1961) *The Coming of the Welfare State*, London: Batsford.

Care in the Community. A Consultative Document on Moving Resources for Care in England. HC(81)9/LAC(81)5, London: DHSS.

Clarke, J., Cochrane A., and Smart, C. (1987) *Ideologies of Welfare*, London: Hutchinson.

Cohen, S. (1971) *Images of Deviance*, Harmondsworth: Penguin.

Cohen, S. and Taylor L.J. (1972) *Psychological Survival: The experience of long-term imprisonment*, Harmondsworth: Penguin.

Declaration on the Rights of the Mentally Retarded Persons (1971). Geneva: United Nations.

Driedger, D. (1989) *The Last Civil Rights Movement*, London: Hurst and Co., New York: St Martins Press.

European Convention on Human Rights (1950), Council of Europe.

Garfinkel, H. (1967) *Studies in Ethnomethodology*, New Jersey: Prentice-Hall.

Goffman, E. (1961) *Asylums*, New York: Anchor.

Health Service Development (1983) Care in the Community and Joint Finance, HC(83)6, LAC(83)5, London: DHSS.

Health and Welfare: The Development of Community Care (1963), Cmnd. 1973, London: HMSO.

International Covenant on Civil and Political Rights (1966) quoted in 'Human Rights and People with a Mental Handicap' M. Gunn, in *Mental Handicap*, vol. 14, September 1986.

Kesey, K. (1962) *One Flew over the Cuckoo's Nest*, London: Methuen.

Laing, R.D. (1964) *Sanity, Madness and the Family*, London: Tavistock.

Lemert, E. (1967) *Human Deviance, Social Problems and Social Control*, New Jersey: Prentice-Hall.

Meade, G.H. (1934) *Mind, Self and Society*, Chicago: University of Chicago Press.

Morris, T., and P. (1963) *Pentonville*, London: Routledge and Kegan Paul.

O'Brien, J. (1987) *A Framework for Accomplishment*, Decatur USA: Responsive Systems Associates.

Parsons, T. (1951) *The Social System*, Glencoe, USA: The Free Press.

Report of the Royal Commission on Mental Illness and Mental Deficiency (1957), Cmnd. 169, London: HMSO.

Robb, B. (1967) *Sans Everything*, London: Methuen.

Szasz, T. (1962) *The Myth of Mental Illness*, New York: Harper and Row.

Universal Declaration of Human Rights (1948), Geneva: United Nations.

Wolfensberger, W. (1972) *The Principle of Normalization in Human Services*, Syracuse: Human Policy Press.

Wolfensberger, W., and Glenn, S. (1975) *PASS 3: Program Analysis of Service Systems*, handbook, 3rd Edition, Toronto: National Institute on Mental Retardation.

Wolfensberger, W., and Thomas, S. (1983) *PASSING: Program Analysis of Service Systems Implementation of Normalization Goals*, Toronto: National Institute on Mental Retardation.

5 Normalisation and applied behaviour analysis

Values and technology in human services[1]

Peter McGill and Eric Emerson

Conflicts between normalisation and applied behaviour analysis are, in part, related to the relative emphases they lay on values and technology. While normalisation has primarily offered a system of values to underpin human services, applied behaviour analysis has focused on the development and implementation of an effective technology of intervention. This chapter explores the possibilities for using applied behaviour analysis within the normalisation framework and of viewing normalisation from the relative clarity of a behavioural perspective.

Applied behaviour analysis has its roots in the behaviourism of B.F. Skinner. Skinner was responsible for two main developments, one scientific and one philosophical. His scientific work (for example, Skinner 1938; Ferster and Skinner 1957), which became known as the experimental analysis of behaviour, studied the behaviour of animals under controlled laboratory conditions and codified the principles to emerge from that study. The most important of these related to the effects of immediate consequences of behaviour in either increasing (reinforcing) or decreasing (punishing) the future probability of the behaviour occurring. In addition, these experimental studies drew attention to the importance of the immediate antecedents of behaviour in setting the occasion for behaviour to occur by virtue of their previous association with reinforcing or punishing consequences. These basic principles have been considerably elaborated and extended by the work of Skinner and others. Today the discipline continues to seek further elaboration through the study of both animal and human behaviour (Lowe *et al.* 1985).

Skinner's second contribution was radical behaviourism which he has described as the philosophical interpretation of the science of behaviour (Skinner 1974). Going beyond existing knowledge, Skinner extrapolated the basic principles of behaviour discovered from experimental studies to the interpretation of complex human behaviour (Skinner 1953) and to speculate in particular, about the roles served by language (Skinner 1957) and cognition (Skinner 1985).

Since the late 1940s and with increasing momentum, the discipline of applied behaviour analysis has sought to apply these basic principles to socially important problems. Initially, work focused on the behaviours of people who had been discounted by society as unable or unwilling to change. Thus early work with people with learning difficulties showed that their behaviour was indeed open to change and was sensitive to the systematic alteration of environmental antecedents and consequences (for example, Fuller 1949; Wolf *et al.* 1964). Similarly, Ayllon and Azrin's (1968) famous study of token economy demonstrated the potential for change amongst people with mental health problems who had, in effect, been abandoned by society. These and subsequent demonstrations (for example, Bellamy *et al.* 1979; Gold 1975) have had a significant impact and led to a reassessment of what achievements may be possible for people with severe disabilities.

The success of this approach led to its increasing use and in the late 1960s, it was formalised as a discipline. The *Journal of Applied Behavior Analysis* was first published in 1968 and in its first volume, Baer *et al.* (1968) provided an account of the nature of applied behaviour analysis as it ought to be practised. They suggested (cf. Baer *et al.* 1987) that applied behaviour analytic studies should be:

- *Applied*: In that the behaviours and events studied should be of importance to society.
- *Behavioural*: In that studies should be concerned with what people do.
- *Analytic*: In that studies should provide a 'believable demonstration of the events that can be responsible for the occurrence or non-occurrence of' the behaviour, usually by the demonstration of experimental control.
- *Technological*: In that techniques used are identified and described in a manner that allows replication.
- *Conceptually Systematic*: In that the procedures used are shown to be relevant to basic behavioural principles.
- *Effective*: In that socially significant changes in behaviour are achieved.
- *General*: In that the behavioural change 'proves durable over time . . . appears in a wide variety of possible environments or . . . spreads to a wide variety of related behaviours'.

Since 1968, the practice of applied behaviour analysis has steadily advanced both in its traditional areas of application and in many new fields (Cullen 1988). Work in the field of learning difficulties has focused on approaches to the development of competence and the reduction of challenging behaviour (for example, Bailey *et al.* 1987). Many studies have demonstrated the success of the approach in teaching skilled behaviour to people with severe learning difficulties (for example, Azrin and Armstrong 1973; O'Neil and Bellamy 1978), and increasingly, techniques are being developed which stress the generalised use of these skills in everyday life (for example, Callahan 1985; Horner *et al.* 1988). The management of challenging behaviour has been transformed by the development of approaches which have been effective with people who have shown aggressive (Danforth and Drabman 1989), self-injurious (Schroeder *et al.* 1981) and stereotyped behaviours (Koegel and Koegel 1989).

Applied behaviour analysis has also made significant contributions to other fields including: the rehabilitation of people with chronic psychiatric disorder or acquired brain damage (Paul and Lentz 1977; Wood and Eames 1981); the treatment of delinquent children and adolescents (Fixsen *et al.* 1973) and the treatment of individuals (Schwartz and Goldiamond 1975), couples (Azrin *et al.* 1973), families (Patterson and Reid 1973) and organisations (Davey 1981) whose behaviour is defined by themselves or others as dysfunctional.

Applied behaviour analysis has also been increasingly used in addressing social rather than purely clinical problems, for example: to promote seat belt usage (Williams *et al.* 1989); to reduce smoking (Stitzer *et al.* 1986) or other forms of substance abuse (McCaul *et al.* 1984); to promote environmentally sound behaviour (Winett *et al.* 1985). More recently, attention has come to focus upon the application of behaviour analysis to societal and cultural problems such as unemployment and law enforcement (for example, Malagodi 1986; Malagodi and Jackson 1989; Sidman 1989).

The concern of applied behaviour analysis with environmental antecedents and consequences has significant implications for its wider application. The prescription of medication or psychotherapy does not usually carry with it any requirement to alter aspects of the individual's everyday environment. In contrast, applied behaviour analysis by definition can only be successful in bringing about behavioural changes if it succeeds in altering the social and physical environments to which individuals are exposed. Much early work in applied behaviour analysis failed to attend to the systemic implications of this requirement (Holland 1978). As a result, there were many demonstrations of highly effective interventions carried out under carefully controlled conditions, but far fewer examples of the maintenance and generalisation of behavioural change within the natural environment.

This concern with sustaining socially significant changes has led applied behaviour analysis in the direction of attempting to change the design, organisation and operation of services (for example, Jenkins *et al.* 1987;

Parsons *et al.* 1989). In addressing this task, applied behaviour analysis has had to engage with ideologies about service design which derive from quite different schools of thought. In the field of learning difficulties in particular, the most significant competing agenda has been normalisation (Wolfensberger 1972, 1980a; Wolfensberger and Glenn 1975; Wolfensberger and Thomas 1983) and social role valorisation (Wolfensberger 1983a).

In this chapter we will attempt to examine some of the points of correspondence and conflict between these two approaches. First, we will address the nature and possible sources of the apparent conflict between normalisation and applied behaviour analysis. In the second part of the chapter, we will examine a basis for a possible *rapprochement* and identify the contributions that each approach may make to the other. While this analysis is perhaps most pertinent to the field of learning difficulties, many of the issues are likely to carry more general implications. Accordingly, while the majority of our illustrations will come from learning difficulties we will include, where appropriate, examples drawn from work with other client groups. It should also be noted that the analysis relates specifically to the relationship between applied behaviour analysis and Wolfensberger's formulations of normalisation. The relationship between applied behaviour analysis and other formulations of normalisation (cf. Emerson, this volume) will not be explored in any detail.

THE NATURE AND SOURCES OF THE CONFLICT BETWEEN NORMALISATION AND APPLIED BEHAVIOUR ANALYSIS

Significant proponents of both applied behaviour analysis (for example, Marchetti and Matson 1981; Mulick and Kedesdy 1988) and normalisation (for example, Wolfensberger 1989) have questioned the value of the 'other' approach. Similar concerns have been voiced by practitioners allied with one or other field (for example, Baldwin 1989; Walker 1987).

The most common criticisms of normalisation have reflected concerns that normalisation either: (1) advocates intervention strategies that have been insufficiently validated (Baldwin 1985, 1989; Mesibov 1976; Throne 1975) or which are even potentially counterproductive (Mulick and Kedesdy 1988); or (2) is equivalent to a policy of non-intervention (Aanes and Haagenson 1978; Clifford 1984). For example, Marchetti and Matson (1981) suggest that

> the minimal amount of experimental data that is available does not support the applicability of *non-specific treatments* such as normalisation, which *basically consists of community placement with a de-emphasis on formalised training.*
>
> (Marchetti and Matson 1981: 212, emphasis added)

Criticisms of applied behaviour analysis, on the other hand, have tended to reflect a belief that it represents a dehumanising technology for the repressive social control of devalued persons (Cohen 1985; Lovett 1985; McGee *et al.* 1987; Wolfensberger 1989). Wolfensberger (1989) also rejects applied behaviour analysis on the grounds that it:

(1) is tied to a materialistic ideology which treats people as machines whose behaviour can be conceived of as separate unintegrated bits;
(2) is applied in a displaced and disembodied fashion with interventions failing to consider the causes or context of behaviour;
(3) is applied as a substitute for the provision of normative life conditions;
(4) is based upon empirical evidence of short-term successes which disguise long-term failure really to change the lives of service users.

In order to understand the conflict between these two approaches, it is necessary to understand their respective scientific ideologies and the nature of their implementation in human services. First, comparison of the philosophical roots of applied behaviour analysis and normalisation reveals some important divisions. Three key differences are particularly significant: the relative importance each approach attaches to empiricism and theory building; the breadth of conceptualisation of the two models; and methodological differences between the approaches with respect to the notion of 'acceptable' evidence.

Normalisation reflects a diversity of influences. Important in this context, however, is the foundation of normalisation on societal reaction or labelling theories of deviance (Burton 1983; Flynn and Nitsch 1980; Wolfensberger 1972). Societal reaction theory suggests that deviant behaviour can largely be accounted for by looking at the ways in which society responds to people labelled as deviant (secondary deviation). Much less importance is attached to any impairment or difference (primary deviation) which may have originally led to the individual becoming so labelled in the first place. The idea that deviance is caused by society's oppressive response to people who were unfortunate enough to be labelled gained ready acceptance in the 1960s and 1970s (for example, Rosenhan 1973; Scheff 1966; Whitehead, this volume).

With respect to the field of learning difficulties, labelling came to serve as 'a nice catchall phrase to explain anything relative to mental retardation' (Rowitz 1974: 265). There is little empirical support, though, for such 'strong' versions of labelling theory either with respect to learning difficulties (for example, Gordon 1975; Guskin 1978) or mental health (for example, Gove 1975, 1982). This is not to deny the fact that considerable evidence exists to suggest that society's response to people with learning difficulties or mental health problems is likely to be unhelpful, if not downright damaging (for example, Link 1982; Link *et al.* 1989; Oswin 1978; Repp *et al.* 1987). It does, however, question the adequacy of societal reaction theory in providing a comprehensive explanation of 'deviant' behaviour.

Because it is based upon societal reaction theory, normalisation shares many of its key attributes (Scull 1984) including:

- a social-psychological orientation which stresses such issues as attitude formation, stereotyping, symbolic marking and stigma in accounting for both deviant behaviour (Jacobsen 1989; Wolfensberger 1989) and social or institutional responses to devalued groups (cf. Wolfensberger 1975);
- a denial, or at least failure to attend to, the importance of people's real impairments;
- a tendency to romanticise deviant behaviour (for example, Wolfensberger 1988a); and
- a reliance upon qualitative methods in what little research the approach appears to have generated (for example, Bercovici 1983; Ward 1988).

These tendencies have resulted in normalisation focusing upon the avoidance or reversal of common processes in the social creation of deviance (for example, the segregation, congregation and symbolic marking of members of deviant groups).

Applied behaviour analysis represents a marked contrast in approach. Its grounding in Skinner's behaviourism is reflected in its emphasis on empiricism, an abhorrence of theory building and a focus upon the quantitative analysis of the behaviour of individuals. This has often resulted in behaviour analysts focusing upon ameliorating the impact of people's impairments through, for example, the development of powerful teaching technologies. Unfortunately, such efforts have rarely been linked to systematic attempts to analyse the role of wider social processes in creating or sustaining deviant behaviour. This failure has, in turn, provided fertile ground for those wishing to equate applied behaviour analysis with coercive social control.

In many ways, the conflict between these two approaches bears a closer relationship to these underlying ideological and epistemological differences than to any of the specific objections raised. The conflict has been fuelled, however, by their impact on human services. While both approaches have influenced the way in which we talk about the aims and design of services, their actual application has proven to be simplistic and sporadic (for example, Cullen 1988; Flynn 1980; Michael 1980; Stolz 1981), an outcome which perhaps reflects the depth of devaluation of human service users in our society (Holland 1978). With respect to applied behaviour analysis, LaVigna and Donnellan (1986) point out that

> some of the greatest abuses against learners in our mental health/ education delivery systems come not from inappropriate utilization of behavioral intervention but from the lack of application of such techno- logy in situations that clearly warrant it.
>
> (LaVigna and Donnellan 1986: 12)

Similarly, services have largely failed to implement practices and proce- dures derived from normalisation. Wolfensberger (1989) argues that the embracing of normalisation by human services is more rhetoric than reality.

In many ways it appears that the main influence exerted on services by *both* approaches has been purely symbolic. That is, their 'implementation' has largely consisted of the relabelling and legitimisation of existing proce- dures in new terminologies. Thus, degrading and abusive reward and punishment regimes have become 'habilitative behavioural interventions', punitive seclusion has become 'time-out' and the dumping of people into 'the community' has come to exemplify 'the dignity of risk' (see Baker 1983; Wolfensberger 1980a: 101–5). In general, services have placed little emphasis on the implementation of empirically validated methods for enhancing the personal competence of service users, have disguised in- action by a fog of high-sounding rhetoric and all too often have used normalisation as justification for *laissez-faire* and/or punitive approaches which meet service rather than client needs.

Indeed, Wolfensberger's (1989) criticisms of applied behaviour analysis can be seen as criticisms of the faulty or incomplete implementation of the approach rather than of its integral features. There is, for example, no doubt that the *practice* of applied behaviour analysis has often failed adequately to consider the ecological context within which an individual is behaving; has sought to intervene without due attention to the root causes of a phenomenon (in behavioural terms, without completing an adequate func- tional analysis) and has been much more energetic in attending to the short- rather than the long-term effects of its interventions (Baer *et al*. 1987; Hayes *et al*. 1980; Michael 1980).

As noted above, these 'perversions' of *both* approaches have provided further evidence to support people's misconceptions (for example, Clifford 1984). In another sense, however, both approaches have served to provide intellectual camouflage for the implementation of often repressive social policies.

POSSIBILITIES FOR *RAPPROCHEMENT*

Applied behaviour analysis can be characterised as a technology bereft of any inherent guiding principles regarding either goal selection or procedural acceptability. Normalisation, on the other hand, represents a value-laden conceptual framework bereft of a systematic technology for effecting behaviour change. Viewed in such a manner the possibility of some degree of *rapprochement* seems clear.

Such a possibility has indeed, been proposed before. In an earlier formulation of normalisation, Wolfensberger (1972: 131) suggested that 'operant shaping . . . is an approach of vast potential' that 'could be massively injected into our service systems', though it is clear from his later writings (for example, Wolfensberger 1989) that his views on this topic have changed somewhat. Roos (1972) and Flynn and Nitsch (1980) have also both addressed the reconciliation or *rapprochement* of behavioural theory and normalisation. Enhancing the personal competencies of devalued people and reducing their devaluing characteristics remain as fundamental aims of normalisation (Wolfensberger and Thomas 1983) and applied behaviour analysis (Baer *et al*. 1968).

Attempts at *rapprochement*, however, cause considerable difficulties. As we have argued above, applied behaviour analysis and normalisation reflect markedly divergent scientific traditions. In addition, their (mis)application in human services has fuelled criticisms by their opponents, who have confused customary practices with basic conceptions. In the following discussion, we consider in detail the implications and possibilities of such a *rapprochement*.

THE IMPLICATIONS OF *RAPPROCHEMENT* FOR APPLIED BEHAVIOUR ANALYSIS

If a process of *rapprochement* were to be pursued how would theory, practice and research in applied behaviour analysis change? Two major implications are immediately apparent. First, applied behaviour analysis would need to develop methods for the assessment of the procedures and goals of interventions in terms of the former's cultural value and the latter's contribution to supporting people in valued social roles. Second, behaviour analysts would need to consider the contribution of normalisation in setting some of the agenda for the development of behavioural theory and practice, particularly in relation to expanding its therapeutic focus from the behaviour of the individual to analysis of and intervention with the cultural and social systems of which they are part.

The need for applied behaviour analysis to attend to the social accept-ability of intervention procedures is becoming increasingly apparent. Many instances can, of course, be found in which applied behaviour analysis is not used in a valued way. For example, applied behaviour analysis has shown an unwarranted reliance on the use of punitive methods for reducing the severity of challenging behaviours shown by people with learning difficulties (for example, Lennox *et al.* 1988; Lundervold and Bourland 1988). Most people would probably agree that shocking people with cattle prods (Carr and Lovaas 1983) or filling their mouths with aerosol shaving cream (Conway and Butcher 1974) or tabasco sauce (Altmeyer *et al.* 1985) is inconsistent with the requirements of normalisation to use procedures that enhance the social image of service users. Indeed, Wolfensberger (1988b) has suggested that the failure of behaviour analysts to 'take the image dimension seriously enough, if they take it seriously at all' is one of the key areas in which behaviour analysts clash with normalisation.

While we would not advocate such interventions it should be pointed out that, in so far as self-injurious behaviour is reduced, they are powerful techniques to remove devaluing characteristics. The outcome is consistent with normalisation, though the method used is clearly not. This conflict within normalisation highlights the multifaceted nature of the approach. Indeed, Wolfensberger (1980a) argues that it is to be expected that different corollaries of normalisation will often conflict with each other when applied to specific situations.

Attending to the broader social impact of intervention procedures would sometimes result in decisions to forego the most powerful intervention, that is, to select a procedure which may not be the most effective in bringing about behaviour change but is preferable on the grounds of cultural values. Behaviour analysts are familiar with the notion that immediate clinical effects are a necessary *but not sufficient* condition for choosing an effective intervention. Willems (1974) pointed to the frequent failure of behaviour analysis to attend to its unintended social consequences and called for the collection of information about the effects of interventions over longer time-frames and with regard to a wider range of implications for people's lives. This attempt by applied behaviour analysis to address the broader social impact of its activities is reflected in the development of techniques of social validation (Baer *et al.* 1987; Kazdin 1977; Kazdin and Matson 1981; Wolf 1978) which have been concerned to investigate the social acceptability of treatment procedures, the social importance of treatment goals and the degree of subjective satisfaction with treatment outcomes. At present, however, the technology of social validation is rather crude (Baer *et al.* 1987) and the approach assumes (probably erroneously) that the personal values of private citizens provide a useful measure of cultural value and that lay people are able to make correct technical judgements about the effectiveness of a particular intervention (Schwade 1979). Flynn and Nitsch (1980) pointed to the possible value of *rapprochement* in strengthening behaviour analysts' concern with social validity. An example is provided by Brown (1988) who outlines a procedure for assessing teaching goals against O'Brien's (1987) notion of service accomplishments. This enables direct care workers to evaluate the social relevance and appropriateness of the skills which they are teaching people with learning difficulties.

Methods for assessing behavioural procedures and goals with respect to their social and cultural value are unlikely to be simple, especially in view of the multifaceted nature of normalisation. Judgements will inevitably be relative rather than absolute and there are likely to be many genuinely difficult conflicts and 'trade-offs' to be made. What do we do, for example, if a person with a psychiatric label chooses to spend all their time in their bedroom, thus defeating the service's efforts to engage them in activities which will promote independence and integration? To what extent should we make potential reinforcers, such as attention, food and drink, contingent on the person's participating in such activities? Normalisation provides a framework for analysing these issues and makes some suggestions about resolution (see Emerson, this volume).

The second main implication of *rapprochement* would be that applied behaviour analysis would need to address the propositions derived from normalisation. Normalisation attaches great importance to phenomena such as expectation and labelling, processes which are not behaviourally well-defined. This has often led to their rejection by behaviour analysts as hypothetical variables unamenable to behavioural investigation. However, Skinner (1953) suggests that clinical, sociological and anthropological observations can often form the basis for more systematic, experimental investigations. Such investigations should define concepts such as 'expectations' in behavioural terms and investigate the circumstances governing their occurrence and influence. There may remain some conflict between the apparently internal account favoured by normalisation (expectations are perceived as things which we 'carry around' in our heads) and the external account sought by applied behaviour analysts, although the development of interest by behaviour analysis in rule-governed behaviour (for example, Blakely and Schlinger 1987; Hayes 1990) and behavioural ecology (for example, Rogers-Warren and Warren 1977; Schroeder 1990) could point to fruitful areas of collaboration.

In practice, then, *rapprochement* would support and hopefully accelerate movement in directions already being taken by behaviour analysis. The influence of normalisation would be likely to lead to the increased use of non-aversive, constructional methods for behaviour change within a broader ecological framework.

Schwartz and Goldiamond (1975) suggest that on grounds of both effectiveness and ethics, behaviourism should adopt a constructional approach to problem behaviour. Whereas a pathological approach concentrates on the elimination of difficult behaviours, a constructional approach seeks to build up a repertoire of positive alternatives. For example, a constructional approach to self-injurious behaviour would involve an initial analysis of the functions served by the behaviour (for example, to gain attention, to avoid demands) followed by teaching the person to use alternative ways of obtaining such consequences, alternatives which do not have the physically and socially damaging side-effects of self-injurious behaviour. Such an approach is exemplified in Carr and Durand's (1985) demonstration of the impact of communication training in reducing behaviour problems in child- ren with severe learning difficulties. Parallel developments are also evident in LaVigna and Donnellan's (1986) attempt to outline a variety of non- aversive procedures for helping people overcome challenging behaviours and demonstrate how applied behaviour analysis can take means as well as ends into account in developing effective programmes. Perhaps the clearest example of the probable impact of *rapprochement* is provided in the work of Marc Gold (for example, Callahan 1985; Gold 1975, 1980). Gold uses procedures predominantly drawn from applied behaviour analysis in the context of a philosophy which, like normalisation, stresses the social origins and consequences of diagnostic labels and the need for teaching and intervention to be explicitly valuing of the client.

THE IMPLICATIONS OF *RAPPROCHEMENT* FOR NORMALISATION

If a process of collaboration were to be pursued how would the theory and practice of normalisation change? Four major implications are immediately apparent. First, proponents of normalisation would need to clarify its empirical, theoretical and ideological components. Second, normalisation would benefit from incorporating behavioural concepts into its practice, particularly in relation to the analysis of issues of choice, coercion and control. Third, theoreticians could usefully employ behavioural concepts to clarify the notion of 'values'. Fourth, trainers would benefit from reviewing the methods used in disseminating normalisation.

Normalisation was originally described by Wolfensberger (1972) as an ideology which was based on, and consistent with, the research literature but also included material derived from personal beliefs rather than existing knowledge. More recently, however, he has claimed that normalisation is 'a theoretical system . . . in which there are really very few bits and pieces that do not have extensive empirical support' (Wolfensberger 1989: 181). Clearly, approaches to the design and operation of services need to be able to go beyond existing knowledge. Applied behaviour analysis is, however, a strongly empirical approach and likely to react antithetically to the mixture of empiricism, theory and ideology present in Wolfensberger's writings. If normalisation is to aim for alignment with applied behaviour analysis, one of its first tasks must be to sort out the data from the theory from the ideology. This would clarify the areas in which an experimental analysis could contribute to normalisation and, of equal importance, build up a scientific basis which would serve to protect normalisation from its ideological opponents. Wolfensberger's recent claim regarding the extent of existing empirical support for normalisation (Wolfensberger 1989) has to be viewed in the context of a rather lax approach to notions of credible evidence (cf. Wolfensberger 1980b).

This unscrambling of normalisation may well leave it advocating procedures which are not empirically validated (see Szivos, this volume). This is acceptable so long as it is clear on what basis they are being advocated and that initiatives are evaluated from an open-minded stance, not a rigid moralistic orthodoxy.

The use of normalisation to bring about individual behaviour change could be markedly strengthened in three ways by the incorporation of a behaviour analytic framework. First, a number of recent approaches for the assessment of, and intervention with, individuals have been developed which are clearly based on normalisation principles (for example, Brost *et al.* 1982; O'Brien 1987). These could usefully incorporate some of the concepts and procedures developed by behaviour analysts. For example, Brost *et al.*'s 'Getting to Know You' manual contains procedures for developing a service plan around the particular needs of individual service users. Its methodology is essentially that of participant observation and its results qualitative rather than quantitative. Without discarding this method or the information it generates, applied behaviour analysis would suggest the use of quantitative recording of behaviour as an additional means of gaining useful and reliable information about the person. In addition, the use of behavioural concepts to organise some of the information gained would prove of considerable value.

Second, a behaviour analytic framework could usefully inform practice in relation to enhancing the personal competency and social image of service users. Normalisation already uses some specific behavioural techniques such as 'modelling' and 'behaviour shaping' along with more global or holistic environmental manipulations to bring about behaviour change

(Wolfensberger 1972; Wolfensberger and Thomas 1983). The latter include such strategies as altering the physical settings or client groupings around which a service is based (cf. Wolfensberger and Thomas 1983). Behaviour analysis could helpfully replace normalisation's disembodied eclecticism with a coherent and systematic framework which would be of considerable value to practitioners in defining the conditions under which both specific techniques and more global changes are likely to achieve the desired aims (cf. Flynn and Nitsch 1980).

Third, applied behaviour analysis could help significantly in the analysis of issues surrounding choice and control. Nirje's concept of normalisation (for example, Nirje 1972) and O'Brien's concept of service accomplishments (for example, O'Brien 1987) propose maximising the service user's choice and control over his or her own life. Applied behaviour analysis, being an essentially deterministic discipline, assumes that people may feel free but that this is an illusion concealing the existence of subtly controlling environmental contingencies (cf. Skinner 1971). In line with normalisation, services may substitute constructional for aversive interventions and thus appear to be no longer controlling their clients. In fact, control is still being exerted and may be all the more dangerous for being more subtle.

A common dilemma for normalisation arises when a service user chooses to do something likely to damage their image or competence. Partly, this difficulty reflects a belief that the client has made a free choice which should therefore be respected. Applied behaviour analysis suggests that closer examination will reveal that this choice is not free but arises, for example, through a lack of alternatives from which to choose or a history of being reinforced for displaying unusual or bizarre behaviour. The appropriate course of action involves providing as culturally valued conditions as possible under which different choices might be made. Accepting a choice as free when it is actually under the control of past influences which may have been coercive and constraining does not seem consistent with the broader conception of normalisation or the commitment to offering people with disabilities a new start.

The degree to which client choice can be determined and should be respected is a central issue in 'consent to treatment'. Consent to treatment has generally been considered in terms of the understanding of information provided about the nature and direct consequences of treatment, and the giving of verbal or written permission for the treatment to occur. As a result, difficulties have arisen with certain individuals where these conditions can apparently not be met. It may be the case, for example, that some people with severe learning difficulties cannot understand the nature of the treatment and may not be able to speak or write. Similarly, people who are temporarily in a state of great mental distress may give permission for treatment although they have understood little of the information provided. A third group of people who raise difficulties are those who clearly understand the nature of the treatment and its consequences and are able to give verbal or written permission but who consistently refuse to give such permission and are perceived, because of a lack of treatment, to be a danger to others.

As Goldiamond (1974) points out it is inappropriate to see consent as primarily about the signing of a piece of paper. Consent refers rather to two things – consenting behaviour (actually going along with the treatment procedure) and the conditions under which the consenting behaviour occurs. Consent may, then, be said to have been given when a person goes along with the treatment under conditions that are not coercive. Typical conditions, though, may well be coercive. For example, an individual may consent to a programme of treatment on the promise of earlier discharge from a penal or psychiatric establishment; in these cases, the signing of a consent form is something of an irrelevance. The contingencies applied to the person essentially coerce him or her into going along with the treatment. This is true even if the treatment has directly beneficial consequences for the person; the essential reason for their co-operation is still the probability of earlier discharge. The crucial issue here is the extent to which the consequences of consenting to treatment are treatment-specific, i.e. natural consequences of receiving treatment, rather than affecting the probability of other reinforcers.

The determination of 'informed consent' may then require an analysis of the contingencies applying to the service user. The following discussion, informed by Goldiamond (1974), attempts to characterise the outcomes of such an analysis:

(1) *Consent.* Consent refers to the situation where the consequences of going along with the treatment are treatment-specific, for example, medication leading to a reduction in psychotic symptoms. Consent is more obvious, the more options exist for the person. For example, the degree of consent to taking medication can be said to be greater if alternative treatment options exist. A state of receiving no treatment may in itself be aversive and therefore, if only one treatment is offered, the person might be said to be being coerced into accepting it. Note that this point is true even if there are no other effective treatments available.

(2) *Coercion in the guise of consent.* Someone may refuse medication and, subsequently, be offered a positive reinforcer for consenting to treatment. This is the situation which arises in many token economies

where extra privileges are used to maintain the target behaviours, in this case taking one's medicine. As Goldiamond (1974) and Wexler (1973) point out, this immediately raises the question of why these privileges cannot be available in a non-contingent fashion, particularly as the privileges usually include such things as being allowed to watch television, access to which would not normally be denied in everyday life. Positive reinforcement may be more acceptable but is not necessarily less coercive than negative reinforcement (Skinner 1971).

(3) *Explicit coercion.* Medication may be offered to the person and if refused, it may be made clear that continued refusal will lead to the suspension of all other treatment. If under these circumstances the person 'consents' to medication, this is coercion or, as it might more commonly be described, blackmail.

(4) *Enforced treatment.* Socially sanctioned enforcement may be provided particularly with the third group of individuals described above. The use of force and other means of restricting the individual will be allowed and there is no pretence that consent is required or sought.

We would suggest that the above four categories of consent could usefully be combined into two, viz. consent and coercion. Coercion would include categories 2, 3 and 4, thus making the relationship between services and service users rather more clear-cut.

This framework also has implications for Lovett's (1985) call for the process of behavioural change to be based firmly on negotiation with the 'client', with a view to finding 'ways of working honestly and respectfully with others to develop trusting relationships' (ibid.: 133). This is certainly a culturally valued way of working and to be commended on normalisation grounds. The above analysis suggests, however, that we should not delude ourselves into thinking that we are therefore handing control over to the client; we are just as likely to be exerting covert control, albeit hopefully of a benevolent kind. We need to recognise that the predominant mode of relationship between staff and the users of services is one of control and the exercise of power. Staff are the controllers, staff have more power. If the relationship between staff and clients is to be more balanced we need to provide what Skinner (1974) terms 'counter controls' which can be utilised by or on behalf of those who are currently under control. A variety of possible counter controls exist including self-advocacy (Williams and Schoultz 1982) and advocacy (Wolfensberger and Zauha 1973).

At a more theoretical level, behaviourism has contributions to make to an analysis of the *sine qua non* of normalisation – the concept of values. Skinner (1971) has suggested that values are essentially equivalent to rules specifying how reinforcers are to be obtained. What would this mean in the context of normalisation? Normalisation starts from the observation that certain groups of people are devalued. Behaviourally this can be taken to mean that such people get less of the relevant reinforcers and more of the punishers than typical members of society. This is clearly true and can be illustrated by asking non-disabled people how they would feel about having learning difficulties, for example. In our experience, this almost invariably produces a negative response. On further enquiry, people will list both the reinforcers which would be less available, such as money, sex, cars and so on, and the punishers which would increase, such as being stared at or excluded from valued places. Moreover, having links with devalued people can also be less reinforcing and may even be punishing. This is alluded to in Wolfensberger's (1983b) call for voluntary advocates, on the grounds that devalued people need relationships maintained by the usual reciprocity involved, rather than special rewards such as pay.

Normalisation argues for a process of social revaluation. A culturally valued life can be conceptualized as a life in which there is greater access to reinforcers and less exposure to punishers. Essentially this means a change in the contingencies applying to service users. These contingencies can be changed in two ways: by the development of behaviours which take advantage of normative contingencies ('if you can do this job you'll get this wage'); and by the provision of 'gratuitous' reinforcers ('since you are mentally ill you can have this benefit'). Normalisation would reject the latter in favour of the former because, we would suggest, the latter carries with it other less desirable consequences such as the disapproval of typical members of society who are not eligible for the benefit in question.

The use of culturally valued means is advocated by normalisation as one process which will improve the public perception of people with dis-abilities, that is, make them more rewarding to be with or at least less aversive to other people. Behaviourally there are two complementary paths to this end. We can use our understanding of the conditions under which typical members of society will approach and/or interact with others to increase the chances of their so doing with people with disabilities. Normal-isation's attention to the reduction of the symbolic marking and overt labelling of deviant individuals can be seen in this light. We can also attempt to change the conditions, under which interaction occurs, to make it more likely that non-disabled people will include devalued people in their activities. This process of increasing public tolerance of differentness is an oft-ignored corollary of the normalisation approach (Wolfensberger 1972).

Applied behaviour analysis might also contribute to the teaching and dissemination of normalisation. Baldwin (1985) suggests that this process of dissemination has been mishandled, resulting in the ideas of normal-isation being 'rejected by a hostile audience' (ibid.: 138). It is our impression that PASS and PASSING workshops, the dominant mode of normalisation teaching, are successful at producing three kinds of outcomes – people who are 'converted' and gain an almost religious zeal, people who are completely alienated and people (perhaps the bulk of our services' staff) who honestly attempt to implement their partial (mis)understandings (see Tyne, this volume). Even where attitudes are successfully changed there is no necessary accompanying change in behaviour. Given the contribution of applied behaviour analysis to the development of effective procedures for changing behaviour, there seems to be considerable scope for the application of this knowledge to the teaching and dissemination of normalisation. There appears to be a particular need for teachers of normalisation to review their objectives and methods. Trainers need to be clear as to:

- who are the people who need to learn about normalisation?
- what do they need to learn?
- how will their behaviour change when they have learnt it?
- what are the most effective methods for teaching them?

CONCLUDING COMMENTS

We have argued above that *rapprochement* between normalisation and applied behaviour analysis seems likely to be mutually beneficial despite some irreconcilable underlying differences. On this basis we would recom- mend (cf. Emerson and McGill 1989) that in general, practitioners should address the *practical* commonalities between the two approaches rather than continue to develop unhelpful critiques of imperfect implementation. In addition:

- Normalisation can contribute:
  methods of assessing the procedures of behaviour analytic interventions in terms of cultural value and the goals of behavioural programmes as to whether they contribute to valued social roles;
  further impetus to the developing agenda in behavioural theory and practice to expand its focus from the behaviour of individual service users to analysis of and intervention with the social systems of which they are part.
- Applied behaviour analysis can help in:
  clarifying the empirical, theoretical and ideological components of normalisation;
  providing concepts and methods for the development of normalisation's tools for assessment and intervention particularly in relation to the analysis of issues concerning choice and control;
  clarifying, by behavioural 'translation', the concept of values;
  reviewing the methods used to disseminate and teach normalisation.

Whether current conditions are likely to be supportive of such a *rapprochement* is unclear. Indeed, the vehemence with which proponents continue to dismiss the value of each other's approach (for example, Baldwin 1989; Wolfensberger 1989) bodes poorly for the establishment of a culture of reasoned debate. The behaviour of proponents and practitioners allied to both approaches is, of course, primarily regulated by peer rather than user or data influences. *Rapprochement* is only likely when the distinct communities of behaviour analysts and normalisation advocates begin to address these issues internally. While there is some evidence that this process is underway (for example, Callahan 1985; LaVigna and Donnellan 1986) there is still far to go. The costs of failure, however, are considerable.

Without the contribution of applied behaviour analysis, the enhancement of the personal competencies of deviant persons is likely to be significantly impaired which, when combined with the anti-empirical bias of many practitioners, will provide further fuel to non-interventionist misconceptions of normalisation. Without a coherent framework for selecting intervention goals and an increased awareness of the impact of intervention procedures on the social status and 'image' of service consumers, applied behaviour analysis will continue to be troubled by charges of coercive social control. Meanwhile, people who have to utilise our services will continue to be short-changed.

NOTE

1 Portions of this chapter were first published in Emerson, E. and McGill, P. (1989) 'Normalization and applied behaviour analysis: values and technology in services for people with learning difficulties', *Behavioral Psychotherapy* 17, 2: 101–17.

ACKNOWLEDGEMENTS

We are grateful to Chris Cullen for his helpful comments on an earlier version of this chapter. The ideas presented have developed over a number of years and have relied extensively on discussions with colleagues. We are particularly grateful to Mark Feinman, and our colleagues in the Centre for the Applied Psychology of Social Care, for the many contributions they have made in the course of such discussions.

REFERENCES

Aanes, D., and Haagenson, L. (1978) 'Normalization: Attention to a conceptual disaster', *Mental Retardation* 16: 55–6.

78   *Normalisation*

Altmeyer, B.K., Williams, D.E., and Sams, V. (1985) 'Treatment of severe self-injurious and aggressive biting', *Journal of Behavior Therapy and Experimental Psychiatry* 16: 159–67.

Ayllon, T., and Azrin, N.H. (1968) *The Token Economy: A motivational system for therapy and rehabilitation*, New York: Appleton-Century-Crofts.

Azrin, N.H., and Armstrong, P.M. (1973) 'The "mini-meal" – a rapid method for teaching eating skills to the profoundly retarded', *Mental Retardation* 11: 9–13.

Azrin, N.H., Naster, B.J., and Jones, R.C. (1973) 'Reciprocity counselling: A rapid learning-based procedure for marital counselling', *Behaviour Research and Therapy* 11: 365–82.

Baer, D.M., Wolf, M.M., and Risley, T.R. (1968) 'Some current dimensions of applied behavior analysis', *Journal of Applied Behavior Analysis* 1: 91–7.

Baer, D.M., Wolf, M.M., and Risley, T.R. (1987) 'Some still-current dimensions of applied behavior analysis', *Journal of Applied Behavior Analysis* 20: 313–27.

Bailey, J.S., Shook, G.L., Iwata, B.A., Reid, D.H., and Repp, A.C. (1987) *Behavior Analysis in Developmental Disabilities 1968–1985 from the Journal of Applied Behavior Analysis*, Lawrence, KS: Society for the Experimental Analysis of Behavior.

Baker, M. (1983) 'Hunting and fishing in human services', *TIPS* 3: 1–3.

Baldwin, S. (1985) 'Sheep in wolf's clothing: Impact of normalization teaching on human services and service providers', *International Journal of Rehabilitation Research* 8: 131–42.

Baldwin, S. (1989) 'Applied behaviour analysis and normalization: New carts for old horses? A commentary', *Behavioral Psychotherapy* 17: 305–8.

Bellamy, G.T., Horner, R.H., and Inman, D. (1979) *Vocational Habilitation of Severely Retarded Adults: A direct service technology*, Baltimore: University Park Press.

Bercovici, S.M. (1983) *Barriers to Normalization: The restrictive management of retarded persons*, Baltimore: University Park Press.

Blakely, E., and Schlinger, H. (1987) 'Rules: Function-altering contingency-specifying stimuli', *The Behavior Analyst* 10: 183–7.

Brost, M., Johnson, T.Z., Wagner, L., and Deprey, R.K. (1982) *Getting to Know You: One approach to service planning and assessment for people with disabilities*, Madison, WI: Wisconsin Coalition for Advocacy.

Brown, H. (1988) *Bringing People Back Home: Teaching new skills*, Bexhill-on-Sea: South East Thames Regional Health Authority.

Burton, M. (1983) 'Understanding mental health services: Theory and practice', *Critical Social Policy* 7: 54–74.

Callahan, M. (1985) *A Technology Evolves: What happened when 'try another way' met the real world*, New York: Marc Gold and Associates.

Carr, E.G., and Durand, V.M. (1985) 'Reducing behavior problems through functional communication training', *Journal of Applied Behavior Analysis* 18: 111–26.

Carr, E.G., and Lovaas, O.I. (1983) 'Contingent electric shock as a treatment for severe behavior problems', in S. Axelrod and J. Apsche (eds) *The Effects of Punishment on Human Behavior*, New York: Academic Press.

Clifford, L.X. (1984) 'A reaction to "social role valorization"', *Mental Retardation* 22: 147.

Cohen, S. (1985) *Visions of Social Control*, Cambridge: Polity Press.

Conway, J.B., and Butcher, B.D. (1974) 'Soap in the mouth as an aversive consequence', *Behavior Therapy* 5: 154–6.

Cullen, C. (1988) 'Applied behavior analysis: Contemporary and prospective agenda', in G. Davey and C. Cullen (eds) *Human Operant Conditioning and Behavior Modification*, Chichester: Wiley.

Danforth, J.S., and Drabman, R.S. (1989) 'Aggressive and disruptive behavior', in E. Cipani (ed.) *The Treatment of Severe Behavior Disorders: Behavior analysis approaches*, Washington, DC: American Association on Mental Retardation.

Davey, G. (1981) 'Behaviour modification in organizations', in G. Davey (ed.) *Applications of Conditioning Theory*, London: Methuen.

Emerson, E.B., and McGill, P. (1989) 'Normalization and applied behaviour analysis: Values and technology in services for people with learning difficulties', *Behavioral Psychotherapy* 17: 101–17.

Ferster, C.B., and Skinner, B.F. (1957) *Schedules of Reinforcement*, New York: Appleton-Century-Crofts.

Fixsen, D.L., Phillips, E.L., and Wolf, M.M. (1973) 'Achievement place: Experiments in self-government with predelinquents', *Journal of Applied Behavior Analysis* 6: 31–47.

Flynn, R.J. (1980) 'Normalization, PASS and service quality assessment: How normalizing are current human services', in R.J. Flynn and K.E. Nitsch (eds) *Normalization, Social Integration and Community Services*, Austin, TX: Pro-Ed.

Flynn, R.J., and Nitsch, K.E. (1980) 'Normalization: Accomplishments to date and future priorities', in R.J. Flynn and K.E. Nitsch (eds) *Normalization, Social Integration and Community Services*, Austin, TX: Pro-Ed.

Fuller, P.R. (1949) 'Operant conditioning of a vegetative human organism', *American Journal of Psychology* 62: 587–90.

Gold, M. (1975) 'Vocational training', in J. Wortis (ed.) *Mental Retardation and Developmental Disabilities, Vol, VII*, New York: Bruner Mazel.

Gold, M.W. (1980) *Try Another Way: Training Manual*, Champaign, IL: Research Press.

Goldiamond, I. (1974) 'Toward a constructional approach to social problems: Ethical and constitutional issues raised by applied behavior analysis', *Behaviorism* 2: 1–84.

Gordon, R.A. (1975) 'Examining labelling theory: The case of mental retardation', in W.R. Gove (ed.) *The Labelling of Deviance: Examining a perspective*, London: Wiley.

Gove, W.R. (1975) 'Labelling and mental illness: A critique', in W.R. Gove (ed.) *The Labelling of Deviance*, New York: Sage/Wiley.

Gove, W. (1982) 'Labelling theory's explanation of mental illness: An update of recent evidence', *Deviant Behavior* 3: 307–27.

Guskin, S.L. (1978) 'Theoretical and empirical strategies for studying the labelling of mentally retarded persons', in N.R. Ellis (ed.) *International Review of Research in Mental Retardation* 9, New York: Academic Press.

Hayes, S.C. (1990) *Rule-Governed Behavior: Cognition, contingencies and instructional control*, New York: Plenum.

Hayes, S.C., Rincover, A., and Solnick, J.V. (1980) 'The technical drift of applied behavior analysis', *Journal of Applied Behavior Analysis* 13: 275–85.

Holland, J.G. (1978) 'Behaviorism: Part of the problem or part of the solution?', *Journal of Applied Behavior Analysis* 11: 163–74.

80   *Normalisation*

Horner, R.H., Dunlap, G., and Koegel, R.L. (1988) *Generalization and Maintenance: Life-style changes in applied settings*, Baltimore: Paul H. Brookes.
Jacobsen, J.W. (1989) 'Behavior modification and normalization in conflict?', *Mental Retardation* 27: 179–80.
Jenkins, J., Felce, D., Mansell, J., de Kock, U., and Toogood, S. (1987) 'Organising a residential service', in W. Yule and J. Carr (eds) *Behaviour Modification for People with Mental Handicaps* (2nd Edition), Beckenham: Croom Helm.
Kazdin, A.E. (1977) 'Assessing the clinical or applied importance of behavior change through social validation', *Behavior Modification* 1: 427–52.
Kazdin, A.E., and Matson, J.L. (1981) 'Social validation in mental retardation', *Applied Research in Mental Retardation* 2: 39–53.
Koegel, R.L., and Koegel, R.L. (1989) 'Community referenced research on self-stimulation', in E. Cipani (ed.) *The Treatment of Severe Behavior Disorders: Behavior analysis approaches*, Washington, DC: American Association on Mental Retardation.
LaVigna, G.W., and Donnellan, A.M. (1986) *Alternatives to Punishment: Solving behavior problems with non-aversive strategies*, New York: Irvington.
Lennox, D.B., Miltenberger, R.G., Spengler, P., and Erfanian, N. (1988) 'Decelerative treatment practices with persons who have mental retardation: A review of five years of the literature', *American Journal on Mental Retardation* 92: 492–501.
Link, B. (1982) 'Mental patient status, work, and income: An examination of the effects of a psychiatric label', *American Sociological Review* 47: 202–15.
Link, B.G., Cullen, F.T., Struening, E., Shrout, P.E., and Dohrenwend, B.P. (1989) 'A modified labelling theory approach to mental disorders: An empirical assessment', *American Sociological Review* 54: 400–23.
Lovett, H. (1985) *Cognitive Counselling and Persons with Special Needs*, New York: Praeger.
Lowe, C.F., Richelle, M., Blackman, D.E., and Bradshaw, C.M. (1985) *Behaviour Analysis and Contemporary Psychology*, London: Lawrence Erlbaum and Associates.
Lundervold, D., and Bourland, G. (1988) 'Quantitative analysis of treatment of aggression, self-injury, and property destruction', *Behavior Modification* 12: 590–617.
McCaul, M.E., Stitzer, M.L., Bigelow, G.E., and Liebson, I.A. (1984) 'Contingency management interventions: Effects on treatment outcome during methadone detoxification', *Journal of Applied Behavior Analysis* 17: 35–43.
McGee, J.J., Menolascino, F.J., Hobbs, D.C., and Menousek, P.E. (1987) *Gentle Teaching: A non-aversive approach to helping persons with mental retardation*, New York: Human Sciences Press.
Malagodi, E.F. (1986) 'On radicalizing behaviorism: A call for cultural analysis', *The Behavior Analyst* 9: 1–17.
Malagodi, E.F., and Jackson, K. (1989) 'Behavior analysts and cultural analysis: Troubles and issues', *The Behavior Analyst* 12: 17–33.
Marchetti, A., and Matson, J.L. (1981) 'Training skills for community adjustment', in J.L. Matson and J.R. McCartney (eds) *Handbook of Behavior Modification with the Mentally Retarded*, London: Plenum.
Mesibov, G.B., (1976) 'Alternatives to the principle of normalization', *Mental Retardation* 16: 30–2.

Michael, J.L. (1980) 'Flight from behavior analysis', *The Behavior Analyst* 3: 1–21.

Mulick, J.A., and Kedesdy, J.H. (1988) 'Self–injurious behavior, its treatment, and normalization', *Mental Retardation* 26: 223–9.

Nirje, B. (1972) 'The right to self–determination', in W. Wolfensberger (ed.) *The Principle of Normalization in Human Services*, Toronto: National Institute on Mental Retardation.

O'Brien, J. (1987) 'A guide to life style planning: Using the Activities Catalogue to integrate services and natural support systems', in B.W. Wilcox and G.T. Bellamy (eds) *The Activities Catalogue: An Alternative Curriculum for Youth and Adults with Severe Disabilities*, Baltimore: Brookes.

O'Neill, C.T., and Bellamy, G.T. (1978) 'Evaluation of a procedure for teaching saw chain assembly to a severely retarded woman', *Mental Retardation* 16: 37–41.

Oswin, M. (1978) *Children Living in Long-stay Hospitals*, London: Spastics International Medical Publications.

Parsons, M.B., Cash, V.B., and Reid, D.H. (1989) 'Improving residential treatment services: Implementation and norm-referenced evaluation of a comprehensive management system', *Journal of Applied Behavior Analysis* 22: 143–56.

Patterson, G.R., and Reid, J.B. (1973) 'Intervention for families of aggressive boys: A replication study', *Behaviour Research and Therapy* 11: 382–94.

Paul, G.L., and Lentz, R.J. (1977) *Psychosocial Treatment of Chronic Mental Patients: Milieu versus social-learning programs*, Cambridge, Massachusetts: Harvard University Press.

Repp, A.C., Felce, D., and de Kock, U. (1987) 'Observational studies of staff working with mentally retarded persons: A review', *Research in Developmental Disabilities* 8: 331–50.

Rogers-Warren, A., and Warren, S. (1977) *Ecological Perspectives in Behavior Analysis*, Baltimore: University Park Press.

Roos, P. (1972) 'Reconciling behavior modification procedures with the normalization principle', in W. Wolfensberger (ed.) *The Principle of Normalization in Human Services*, Toronto: National Institute on Mental Retardation.

Rosenhan, D.L. (1973) 'On being sane in insane places', *Science* 179: 250–8.

Rowitz, L. (1974) 'A sociological perspective on labelling', *American Journal of Mental Deficiency* 79: 265–7.

Scheff, T.J. (1966) *Being Mentally Ill*, Chicago: Aldine Press.

Schroeder, S.R. (1990) *Ecobehavioral Analysis and Developmental Disabilities: The twenty first century*, London: Springer-Verlag.

Schroeder, S.R., Schroeder, C.S., Rojahn, J., and Mulick, J.A. (1981) 'Self-injurious behavior: An analysis of behavior management techniques', in J.L. Matson and J.R. McCartney (eds) *Handbook of Behavior Modification with the Mentally Retarded*, New York: Plenum.

Schwade, S. (1979) 'The case against social validation', *Behaviorists for Social Action Journal* 1: 11–17.

Schwartz, A., and Goldiamond, I. (1975) *Social Casework: The behavioral approach*, New York: Columbia University.

Scull, A.T. (1984) 'Competing perspectives on deviance', *Deviant Behavior* 5: 275–89.

Sidman, M. (1989) *Coercion and its Fallout*, Boston: Authors Cooperative.

Skinner, B.F. (1938) *The Behavior of Organisms*, New York: Appleton-Century-Crofts.

Skinner, B.F. (1953) *Science and Human Behavior*, New York: MacMillan.
Skinner, B.F. (1957) *Verbal Behavior*, New York: Appleton-Century-Crofts.
Skinner, B.F. (1971) *Beyond Freedom and Dignity*, New York: Knopf.
Skinner, B.F. (1974) *About Behaviourism*, London: Jonathan Cape.
Skinner, B.F. (1985) 'Cognitive science and behaviourism', *British Journal of Psychology* 76: 291–301.
Stitzer, M.L., Rand, D.S., Bigelow, G.E., and Mead, A.M. (1986) 'Contingent payment procedures for smoking reduction and cessation', *Journal of Applied Behavior Analysis* 19: 197–202.
Stolz, S. (1981) 'Adoption of innovations from applied behavioral research: "Does anybody care?" ', *Journal of Applied Behavior Analysis* 14: 491–506.
Throne, J.M. (1975) 'Normalization through the normalization principle: Right ends, wrong means', *Mental Retardation* 13: 23–5.
Walker, M. (1987) 'Just who benefits from behaviourist techniques?', *Community Living* 1: 4.
Ward, L. (1988) 'Developing opportunities for an ordinary community life', in D. Towell (ed.) *An Ordinary Life in Practice*, London: King's Fund.
Wexler, D.B. (1973) 'Token and taboo: Behavior modification, token economies, and the law', *California Law Review* 61: 81–109.
Willems, E.P. (1974) 'Behavioral technology and behavioral ecology', *Journal of Applied Behavior Analysis* 7: 151–65.
Williams, M., Thyer, B.A., Bailey, J.S., and Harrison, D.F. (1989) 'Promoting safety belt use with traffic signs and prompters', *Journal of Applied Behavior Analysis* 22: 71–6.
Williams, P., and Schoultz, B. (1982) *We Can Speak for Ourselves*, London: Souvenir Press.
Winett, R.A., Leckliter, I.N., Chinn, D.E., Stahl, B., and Love, S.Q. (1985) 'Effects of television modelling on residential energy conservation', *Journal of Applied Behavior Analysis* 18: 33–44.
Wolf, M.M. (1978) 'Social validity: The case for subjective measurement or how applied behavior analysis is finding its heart', *Journal of Applied Behavior Analysis* 11: 203–14.
Wolf, M., Risley, T., and Mees, H. (1964) 'Applications of operant conditioning procedures to the behaviour problems of an autistic child', *Behaviour Research and Therapy* 1: 305–12.
Wolfensberger, W. (1972) *The Principle of Normalization in Human Services*, Toronto: National Institute on Mental Retardation.
Wolfensberger, W. (1975) *The Origin and Nature of our Institutional Models*, Syracuse: Human Policy Press.
Wolfensberger, W. (1980a) 'The definition of normalization: Update, problems, disagreements and misunderstandings', in R.J. Flynn and K.E. Nitsch (eds) *Normalization, Social Integration and Community Services*, Austin, TX: Pro-Ed.
Wolfensberger, W. (1980b) 'Research, empiricism and the principle of normalization', in R.J. Flynn and K.E. Nitsch (eds) *Normalization, Social Integration and Community Services*, Austin, TX: Pro-Ed.
Wolfensberger, W. (1983a) 'Social role valorization: A proposed new term for the principle of normalization', *Mental Retardation* 21: 234–9.
Wolfensberger, W. (1983b) *Reflections on the Status of Citizen Advocacy*, Toronto: National Institute on Mental Retardation.

Wolfensberger, W. (1988a) 'Common assets of mentally retarded people that are commonly not acknowledged', *Mental Retardation* 26: 63–70.

Wolfensberger, W. (1988b) 'Letter to authors dated 21/11/88'.

Wolfensberger, W. (1989) 'Self-injurious behaviour, behavioristic responses, and social role valorization: A reply to Mulick and Kedesdy', *Mental Retardation* 27: 181–4.

Wolfensberger, W., and Glenn, S. (1975) *PASS 3: Program Analysis of Service Systems. Handbook and Field Manual* (3rd Edition), Toronto: National Institute on Mental Retardation.

Wolfensberger, W., and Thomas, S. (1983) *PASSING: Program Analysis of Service Systems Implementation of Normalization Goals*, Toronto: National Institute on Mental Retardation.

Wolfensberger, W., and Zauha, H. (1973) *Citizen Advocacy and Protective Services for the Impaired and Handicapped*, Toronto: National Institute on Mental Retardation.

Wood, R., and Eames, P. (1981) 'Application of behaviour modification in the treatment of traumatically brain-injured adults', in G. Davey (ed.) *Applications of Conditioning Theory*, London: Methuen.

6   Inside-out
A psychodynamic approach to normalisation

Helen Smith and Hilary Brown

Experience shows that maintaining change in services to people with disabilities is extremely difficult, no matter which theories of change are employed. Both psychoanalysis and normalisation have been criticised on the grounds that making difficulties and problems explicit is not enough; attention needs to be paid to the conflicts which will ensue when an individual or an organisation attempts to do things differently. Because of this, it is necessary to understand the ways in which institutions functioned to support staff in their task of caring for people and to defend them from the personal stress inherent in such work. If the regimes which we are trying to replace have in fact grown up to provide a structure which contains the anxiety which the work creates, a change of location will not be enough to reform them. It is important, therefore, to focus on what is going on beneath the surface in new services and on the psychological implications for staff of working in community-based projects, especially those influenced by normalisation.

This chapter explores the links between psychodynamic theory and the theory of normalisation and looks at how these two approaches can inform better services for people with disabilities. Both theories are based on key theoretical concepts which have contributed to our understanding of both good and bad practice. Normalisation has analysed the effects on people of using disability services and, to some extent, explains the covert intention behind 'caring' services. A psychodynamic perspective is helpful in exploring the individual psychological consequences for staff of working in these services, and can explain how institutional structures manage and contain caring relationships which are often painful and challenging to workers' competence and integrity. The chapter ends by considering the kind of support and training which must be offered to front line staff if they are to maintain their closeness to service users and contain the conflicts which that commitment creates.

KEY CONCEPTS

The mother of a young woman with severe learning difficulties said 'Sometimes, I look at her and I think how beautiful she would have been', then quickly she corrected herself, 'I mean she is beautiful but . . . ' (quoted in Brown 1987: 167).

The notion of a Freudian slip has passed into popular usage to express those things which we cannot take responsibility for meaning. In his seminal work *The Origin and Nature of our Institutional Models*, Wolfensberger (1975) exposed the imagery and language which surrounds people with disabilities, especially the pervasiveness of images of death and of subhumanness (such a process is closely allied to racism; see Ferns, this volume). Workers were challenged through PASS courses to ask why, for example, posters of anthropomorphised gorillas should so often be seen in new community services – usually featured doing something inappropriate like cleaning their teeth over the toilet bowl or spilling their dinner all over the place? They feature too often for it to be a coincidence, it was asserted, too often for us to overlook what they are saying about how the workers feel about the job they are doing and the people they are caring for. These are feelings which would not be acknowledged in the statements of values of the agency or by individual workers; the meaning of the pictures would shame both and meet with protestations of denial. Making explicit such feelings is a keystone of the normalisation ideology and is seen as the prime motivator of change. As Wolfensberger (1983) states:

> so much of what goes on in human services is very negative because they enact society's real but destructive intentions and/or address needs other than the clients'. Unpleasant realities are apt to be denied and repressed into unconsciousness, especially if they stand in contrast to the higher values and ideals that people consciously profess. Such denial and repression can take place on a systemic (e.g. societal or organisational) level as well as on a personal/individual one. Thus, entire systems, such as service agencies, service professions, service sectors (e.g. mental health), and even entire societies, can be totally unconscious of some of the most important things they are doing.
> Normalisation incorporates the explicit assumption that consciousness is preferable to unconsciousness and that negative feelings and dynamics should and usually have to be made conscious in order to be adaptively addressed.
>
> (Wolfensberger 1983: 25)

Thus normalisation exposed the covert ambivalence behind so-called 'caring' services. Wolfensberger (1975) and later O'Brien (1980), amongst others, traced the content of prejudice and discrimination towards people with disabilities and showed how this is translated into inadequate, even persecutory working practices and service design. But they, and the movement in general, have not dwelt on the origin of these negative feelings or attempted to trace their development in the internal worlds of people who work in services or in the experiences which they bring to the work. They have consistently located the problem in a historical context rather than a personal one.

Psychodynamic theories explore the boundary between what happens in the real world and how this is perceived and encoded in the internal fantasy and emotional life of the individual. The approaches differ in emphasis as to which comes first – whether the individual projects their internal conflicts on to figures in the outside world, thus repeating patterns already within themselves (Klein 1937, 1940) or whether individuals internalise abuse and conflict which they are subjected to in the outside world and re-enact this in fantasy and in later relationships, as a way of getting their experience validated and acknowledged. Miller (1987) describes how individuals displace the violence which has been done to them on to others weaker than themselves. With this in mind, it becomes important to ask why people choose to go into caring jobs and how they are sustained in them. Miller sees a crucial difference between people who are enabled to acknowledge the hurtful or abusive incidents of their childhood and are believed and helped to deal with these, and those who are not and may then re-enact the violence which has been done to them. The former situation can serve as a motivator if a carer is able to identify with a service user and acknowledge a shared history of powerlessness and hurt. If, on the other hand, the staff person remains unconscious of their own past traumas, they are more likely to use the service user as an object on which to replay their own humiliations and inadequacies, however insignificant or trivial these might seem in the adult world.

In both approaches there is the notion of feelings spilling over from one realm to another, of painful issues squashed down until they seep out in everyday actions and of things absorbed in a fragmented way and hurriedly pushed back into the outside world, on to 'them' or 'the services' or 'society' because the resulting conflicts and inconsistencies cannot be contained.

The ideas presented here depend on the use of psychological concepts first expounded by Freud (1901) and developed by Klein (1937, 1940). Our interpretation of Freud is one which takes his notions of unconscious motivation as being a valuable tool in understanding the behaviour of individuals or groups. However, it is Klein, who, in starkly describing the internal world of infancy and how we are thrown back into it at times of stress, illuminates the heightened sense of ambivalence which many human service workers seek to contain.

Klein describes the anxiety of caring for others as being comparable with the conflicts which exist from earliest childhood when, in reality, the child was dependent on another for its survival and was dominated by two opposing sets of feelings, libidinal and aggressive. The infant feels the force of these feelings out of all proportion and believes them to be literally life-giving and death-dealing. She swings between feeling that she can control other people, notably her mother as the source of food, and feeling powerless and hopeless as her needs are unacknowledged or unmet. At the earliest stage, the infant cannot distinguish clearly between herself and others and builds up an inner world peopled by her own impulses (good and bad) and the significant people (objects) in her life. Because of the per-ceived power of the aggressive instinct, the infant's inner world may be felt to be a battleground, containing many people whom she has damaged and who have damaged her. As Menzies (1970) states,

> The atmosphere is charged with death and destruction. This gives rise to great anxiety. The infant fears for the effect of aggressive forces on the people he loves and on himself. He grieves and mourns over their suffering and experiences depression and despair about his inadequate ability to put right their wrongs. He fears the demands that will be made on him for reparation and the punishment and revenge that may fall on him. He fears that his libidinal impulses and those of other people cannot control the aggressive impulses sufficiently to prevent utter chaos and destruction. The poignancy of the situation is increased because love and longing themselves are felt to be so close to aggression. Greed, frus-tration and envy so easily replace a loving relationship. The phantasy world is characterised by a violence and intensity of feeling quite foreign to the emotional life of the normal adult.
>
> (Menzies 1970: 6)

Caring brings back such conflicts because it is often experienced as a battle or competition between carer and cared for – for time, resources or attention – superimposed on a compassionate relationship; love, longing and aggression are, indeed, inextricably entwined. One way in which people avoid the pain of facing up to these conflicting feelings is to project them on to someone else: if it is too terrifying for me to acknowledge that I do not like a particular service user, I can imagine that he doesn't like me and justify my avoidance of him through his dislike. This process is known, in psycho-dynamic terms, as 'projection' and is widely used by individuals and groups as a defence mechanism against internal anxiety and hostility. It is clearly seen in the treatment of people with disabilities who serve as a repository for the projections of individual fears and anxieties. Society's collective intolerance of disability can be understood in terms of the unconscious motivations which govern the behaviour of both individuals and groups. As individuals, we can find contact with 'madness' or difference terrifying, linking us as it does to the turbulence, chaos and violence of our own inner worlds. In order to cope, society has historically 'split off' and controlled people defined as dangerous, sick, incompetent or unpredictable by placing them in institutions where out of sight is, to coin a phrase, out of mind.

In the move to community care (which in itself is motivated in part by reparation for damage that has been done), large institutions are slowly being closed. We have split off the 'bad' bits of the service and located them in hospitals. Staff in the 'old' institutions are left carrying the baggage of a century of institutionalised services as if they were personally responsible – indeed it is usually those with least power who are left to carry most of the blame. Outside in the new services, however, we continue recreating the splits which characterise our internal worlds, joining cliques which use certain techniques or jargon, or advocating a particular approach to the work. What is missing in the community is a replication of two vital functions of institutions: that of providing a repository for collective projections of madness and difference; and an organisational structure that contains the anxiety aroused by caring for people perceived to be 'different'. Little wonder that hospital closures are so controversial and often opposed by relatives, staff and society at large.

It is essential that these two functions are addressed, especially in projects influenced by normalisation which make explicit attempts to dismantle institutional forms of care. If these projects are to succeed they must consciously deal with these intra-psychic defences. The danger is that service users will yet again miss the chance of an ordinary and fulfilled life as powerful, unconscious forces shift social policy back into the cycle of community/institutional/community care that has characterised our services for people with disabilities over the last two hundred years (Allderidge 1979).

Wolfensberger (1983), in looking at why people were institutionalised, defined the unconscious images which have been projected on to people with disabilities, that of menace, objects of dread, burdens of charity or pity, trivial, sick, less than truly human or a commodity to be bought and sold (see Emerson, this volume). For most members of the public, people with disabilities are 'not like us', they are different, living in another world. For staff, of whatever profession, the same feelings can be manifested and they may put on a professional mantle which separates them from their clients/patients, sometimes to the extent that they no longer perceive the common humanity between themselves and the people who use their services. This degree of psychological separation can lead to the abuse that all too often characterises institutions – the daily restriction of choices, the withholding of rights, and verbal, or even physical, abuse. The other side of this coin is to deny difference in our language and service formulations as if its acknowledgment will blow away a fragile pseudo-acceptance which is masking real and feared destructive feelings. Sinason (1986) cites the frequent changes in language used to describe disability as an attempt at cosmetic change, a view echoed in the disability literature (see for example Abberley 1987). This ties in with the notion of passing (Goffman 1961) where the stigmatised individual attempts to pass for normal rather than expose the painful fact of his difference.

These ideas are useful tools in thinking about the prejudice and stigma associated with disability and highlight the fact that there are no easy answers in carrying forward the commitment to better services for people with disabilities. Adherents of normalisation have a particularly delicate path to tread. As we quoted earlier, normalisation started from an explicit commitment that 'consciousness is preferable to unconsciousness and that negative feelings and dynamics should and usually have to be made conscious in order to be adaptively addressed' (Wolfensberger 1983: 25). The commitment to explore and honestly face up to differences between users and non-disabled people has been somewhat obscured by the imperative within normalisation to censor language and imagery. This is a dilemma which will not go away. Services which use normalisation need to be robust enough to take on board the negative feelings which workers have about the work they do. The alternative is to bring in fresh young workers, fire them up with idealism and then watch them leave when they find they can no longer contain the feelings aroused in daily contact with people who are sometimes difficult, boring, dangerous and sometimes lovely, lonely, lively or depressed – in short, human. Because ambivalence is at the root of all human relationships and because service workers relate to people in less than ideal situations and with a half-hearted mandate from society at large, they must be allowed space and freedom from censure in acknowledging how they feel. Unacknowledged feelings will leak out and, under these circumstances, gorillas on the wall are better than people in cages.

INSTITUTIONAL PRACTICE AS A PSYCHOLOGICAL DEFENCE

Thus institutions function in two ways – at a conscious level they function to care for people, while at an unconscious level they serve to protect the public from people whom they perceive to be dangerous or pitiable. There is a constant tension between these two contradictory purposes and history shows how easily human services turn from benevolence to persecution and restriction as this impulse to be rid of people is enacted. Normalisation has been a useful framework to teach service workers about these dynamics and to make clear their role as intermediaries between people with disabilities and the community at large. But services, both old and new, also operate with conflicting values: at a conscious level they make explicit statements of their idealised values while at an unconscious level they operate routines and procedures which treat service users in ways which belie them. Understanding the roots of the subculture which emerges in services and trying to bring it more closely into line with stated philosophy is an important step, and one in which normalisation training has excelled. The notion of model coherency (Wolfensberger 1983) encapsulates this need to reconcile what services say with what they actually do. But the application of normalisation may inadvertently serve to suppress rather than resolve underlying conflicts, if the underlying agenda of institutions, to distance workers from difficult feelings, is never made explicit. In these circumstances, real change will elude even the most optimistic projects.

Menzies (1970), in her seminal work, *The Functioning of Social Systems as a Defence against Anxiety*, looked at how institutions function to contain anxiety for the staff who work within them. Her work is based on a study of the stress experienced by the nursing profession in an acute general hospital. Despite this particular focus, the work is highly relevant to community care as her contention that caring for people arouses very strong and mixed feelings – pity, compassion, guilt, anxiety, hatred, resentment (of patients who arouse these strong feelings), envy of the care given to them – is equally true in disability services. Menzies points out that people are in hospital precisely because they and their carers find it too stressful for them to be at home. Hospitals, then, must be organised to enable staff to cope, both with the stress generated by users and their families and with the internal anxiety and feelings triggered through the act of caring. She describes how these individual, psychological needs of staff lead to the development of collective, socially structured defences, which become apparent in the culture and working practices of the organisation.

In looking for the origins of institutional (mal)practice in terms of unconscious dynamics we have to ask both what it is that such practices protect staff from facing and how they operate to do so. We have identified four powerful needs which staff respond to by creating defensive practices, in spite of their best intentions – the need to avoid painful feelings, the need to diffuse responsibility for difficult decisions, the need to shield themselves from the intensity of demands on their time and energy and their need to evoke a familiar framework which glosses over the lack of true reciprocity in the paid caring relationship.

First, we agree with Ryan (1980) that much of the way we organise the work we do, in new as well as old services, serves to help professionals 'avoid the pain of handicapped people about the lives they have to lead' (p. 28) and of their part in delivering services which contribute to this hurt. More recently Oswin (1984) described the way classic symptoms of distress and depression were overlooked in children with learning difficulties when they had been separated from their parents for respite care. Their 'lost' behaviours were rationalised away as part of their handicapping conditions, rather than acknowledged as normal responses and as indicative of their pain and hurt. Family members are also marginalised by services which focus almost entirely on the life of the person with a disability. Their grieving is ignored and, while they are often exploited as unpaid carers, they are also castigated by innumerable theories which blame them for the situation or for their inability to cope.

For most workers, the core of their work-related anxiety lies in their relationship with individual service users. Menzies noted that one of the prime ways in which the nursing profession protects its members from close relationships with difficult individuals is by preventing contact with the whole person. This is most clearly done through the task-list system whereby the work is organised via tasks to be done rather than people who need care. This practice continues despite innovations such as the nursing process – shifts tend to have clearly defined tasks and staff within those shifts tend still to assign the work so that one nurse does the baths, another the meals, an occupational therapist does craftwork and so on. In this way, workers are blocked from meaningful and prolonged contact with users – contact which would bring them close to people's real and often distressing feelings.

However, workers in services committed to normalisation find it much more difficult to divide the work in this way. Projects are for a small number of people working/living in small units, the very nature of which militates against the splitting of contact between worker and user. The physical size and psychological closeness challenges this particular social defence which is so manifest in institutions. There is also a directive within normalisation which (rightly) identifies this splitting mechanism as a primary factor in the dehumanisation of people with disabilities.

Services also cocoon their workers from pain by desensitising them to the individual issues of each person they care for. Labelling serves to block the development of one-to-one relationships between staff and patients by subsuming the significance of the individual user under a category. This is true in psychiatry where labels, once assigned, often stick for life (people become 'relapsed schizophrenics' or a 'psychotic in remission') and is especially true for people with learning difficulties whose diagnoses may circumscribe every major life decision. Other institutional defences which protect staff from one-to-one contact with users include the over-riding ethic that a professional worker likes and treats all patients the same; conversely, patients themselves are not expected to mind which member of staff is involved with them or even the sex of the individual who offers them very personal care: stating a personal preference for a particular member of staff is often strongly discouraged. Moving staff frequently from ward to ward cuts off significant relationships, and the impersonal standardisation of the physical environment (for example, every ward has the medicine cupboard in the same place) also perpetuates the notion that all users are the same, with little individuality. Normalisation has successfully challenged the value of giving someone a label which says so little about their needs, interests or abilities. A more relevant focus on the *description* of individuals and their circumstances (such as the 'Getting To Know You' assessment, Brost and Johnson 1982), rather than *diagnosis*, has allowed for the development of more appropriate individualised services.

However, even if staff manage to insulate themselves from the pain of others they will still have to face their own anxiety about making mistakes. Workers are faced with immense responsibility in the work they do and many defensive practices and structures develop to shield them from this. Indeed the work, although it is often tedious and repetitive, is always made stressful by the possibility that something awful will happen for which an individual worker would bear the guilt. (In this it is similar to childcare, where similar mechanisms of control and punishment help to contain anxiety in the face of risk.) There are many ways in which institutions protect staff from the anxiety caused by making decisions and taking responsibility; in nursing especially, the number and variety of decisions are minimised through the rituals of nursing tasks. Even with more complex senior roles, efforts are made to standardise performance. Menzies refers to a 'collusive redistribution of responsibility' – a social system of denial and projection which helps staff cope with this tension. She found that more skilled nurses than were necessary were employed to perform simple domestic tasks. The reason given to her for this situation was that junior staff were too irresponsible to do even the simplest thing, a judgement indicative of projection.

In the scandals that have occurred in long-stay institutions, it is junior staff who are most vulnerable to being blamed and indeed it is often their direct care, or lack of it, which has caused the neglect or abuse. In services committed to normalisation, the direct impact of responsibility for service users is hard to evade. This may explain why the issue of responsibility is still so fraught in community services and suggests that the need to diffuse responsibility for decision making through institutional structures remains a strong motivator of individual behaviour. The reason many staff give for not wanting to move into the community is that patients will be put at risk, but when probed it is often their own anxiety which is being voiced. Normalisation clearly states the importance of encouraging users to engage in age-appropriate behaviour and this includes a consideration of what is acceptable risk (see Braisby *et al.* 1988). However, perhaps in an unconscious attempt to avoid responsibility, many new services still operate hierarchically and employ 'qualified' staff to perform tasks which are unrelated to their professional training. The challenge for services operating according to normalisation is to enable both staff and service users to take as much responsibility as they feel able to, supported by consultation and well defined risk-taking procedures.

A third area in which defences arise is as a shield against excessive demands for social interaction or practical or emotional input (excessive being defined differently by different individuals and by the same individuals at different times, depending on their own health and stamina). Morris (1969) observed how hospital workers became obsessed by routine chores, such as counting sheets, and defined them as the core task in preference to relating to service users. It is significant that people with severe and long-term disabilities are less likely to have access to the more skilled workers. Staff on long-stay wards are caring for people with the most complex and demanding needs, yet they tend to be less skilled, less valued and less well paid than their colleagues working in other services, especially the acute sector. Moreover, professionally qualified staff tend to organise their work in terms of short-term interventions and limit their time with people with disabilities through appointments and clinics. It seems that these more skilled workers are able to use their knowledge and status to move away from those people most likely to arouse primitive feelings of powerlessness and helplessness. This leaves workers with the fewest skills working with people who present the greatest challenge to professional and personal competence – it should be no surprise, then, that patterns of care become rigid and inflexible or that advice from these privileged professionals is often perceived as irrelevant or unhelpful.

Lastly, institutional practices are often encapsulated in perversions of other relationships which are used to justify authority and control. Morris (1969) identified three such modes of working in a mental handicap hospital – a 'colonial' mentality, wherein rigid separation between workers and service users was justified, the 'prefect and fag' model, whereby favourites were conscripted to run errands and do chores in return for protection and rewards, and the most usual model of parent/child interactions which characterised most staff attitudes and practices. New services have developed new fictions but these are not necessarily more helpful: they include, for example, the notion of staff as friends or as equal colleagues. Newer rationalisations tend to be more optimistic and more equitable but they also gloss over the professional and probably time-limited commitment inherent in a relationship which is, when all is said and done, just part of the work.

Wolfensberger (1987) asserted that the payment of staff, in and of itself, contributed to the chasm between people with disabilities and their carers and that equality for people with disabilities would never be promoted while care is driven by financial motivation, rather than love and friendship. Following this argument to its limits, he now advocates the abolition of formally organised human services on the assumption that the 'community' will undertake the care of its members. This exhortation for communities to care, however, denies the reality for the vast majority of unpaid carers, most of whom, of course, are women (Finch and Groves 1983; see also Brown and Smith, this volume). Research (Parker 1985) has shown that carers' lives are characterised by poverty, exhaustion through insufficient support, lack of physical aids and inadequate accommodation. His approach glosses over the skills and inner resources which are needed if one is to care for someone whose behaviour is violent, self-injurious or so disturbed that it becomes impossible to understand.

Wolfensberger's stance can also be questioned from a psychodynamic perspective as to whether a notion of unconditional love, that is, a moral imperative to care, is a healthy basis for an adult relationship between cared for and carer. It is neither feasible nor desirable, therefore, to tackle the problems caused through the user/worker divide by simply abolishing paid caring work: unpaid carers face the same stresses, exacerbated by fewer resources and less opportunity to protect and nurture themselves. Nor is it possible to dissolve the divide: workers cannot support someone in achieving independence if there are no boundaries to the care which is offered. Indeed, some people with physical disabilities *prefer* to pay for their care, feeling that this is the only way they can remain in control of their lives. Carers (paid and unpaid) need boundaries which separate them emotionally and physically when caring for individuals. Wolfensberger, in advocating the dismantling of these boundaries, places an unacceptable burden on carers already oppressed through low incomes, low status and lack of recognition.

Good practice lies somewhere between these two extremes and the challenge for new services is to support workers in letting go of the 'task-list' system and encouraging contact with the whole of the person, while at the same time maintaining appropriate boundaries and legitimating periodic relief from the stress of face to face contact. Workers will not be effective if they are overwhelmed by what may be very difficult behaviour to understand or tolerate; however, neither will they be effective if their response is to negate the individual by splitting them into fragmented component tasks. These are not easy issues to get right, but are often crucial in helping users have fulfilled lives in the community.

Thus it is possible to see how practice grows up which enables workers to explain away distress and to distance themselves from their own part in delivering services in order to protect themselves from painful feelings. Elaborate justifications are used to maintain such defences in the face of outsiders or the challenges of new ways of working. Inherent in normalisation is an accurate reversal of the defence mechanisms which characterised institutional life. Smaller staff groups in new projects means there is less scope for the frequent change of staff which occurred in hospital settings, and more personalised living environments ensure that people are seen more in their own right. It is particularly important, therefore, to consider these social defences in relation to normalisation, as the emphasis of normalisation-inspired services on the ordinariness of people who are receiving care and their less rigidly defined service hierarchies may invoke different internal conflicts.

Lamb (1979) has identified how workers in community-based projects can over-identify with users to the extent that users come to play too large a role in validating their own worth. Not recognising this situation, staff can become disillusioned and feel de-skilled when users fail to achieve their (the workers') expectations. The balance which has to be achieved is to recognise the separate identities of worker and service user. This will allow workers to redefine what is a 'success' in work terms and may help protect them from burn-out. Developing *appropriate* relationships with service users will best be facilitated by staff who have a high degree of personal maturity; recruitment and training must take this into account.

If community care is to succeed, the unconscious defences which functioned to contain anxiety in the institution must be replaced or restructured. This does not mean that rigid working practices should be replicated but that their underlying functions be addressed through more positive alternatives. There is evidence that this is beginning to be tackled in job design, the development of risk-taking policies and procedures for consultation and more guidance about *how* to do the work as opposed to simply what it is we are aiming at. Unless these issues are addressed, community services (and particularly services which set out with a strong commitment to normalisation) run the risk of being highly stressful for staff. This may lead to the rebuilding of unconscious defences into the organisational structure of new services, resulting in working practices and attitudes reminiscent of the old institutional regimes or the development of new avenues of avoidance which may be indicated by high staff turnover, reliance on agency staff or staff using normalisation to justify a *laissez-faire* stance which minimises users' real difficulties.

TRAINING AND SUPPORT FOR STAFF

Caring for people is a job which requires a high degree of personal maturation if the task itself and the level of responsibility are to be adequately coped with – yet most training focuses almost entirely on skills and techniques, with minimal emphasis on helping workers mature in the work setting. Little attempt is made to help individuals confront the anxiety-evoking aspects of their work and so develop a personal capacity to cope more effectively with painful conflicts. Despite dealing with very real stress, staff are offered few opportunities to express their own emotional distress or reaction to the work. While traditional services effected this suppression of feelings by laying great emphasis on professional detachment, services committed to normalisation tend to suppress it by accentuating the positive aspects of service users to the exclusion of distress or concerns about their disabilities.

Normalisation projects are rooted in a strong, clear philosophy, yet unless training addresses the psychological issues involved in making this transition, staff can fall into a void between institutional and new ways of working (Kingsley and Smith 1989). Training must pay as much attention to dealing with the anxiety evoked by the work as to practical, working skills. This means developing effective supervision, an emphasis on multi-disciplinary training and a focus on user involvement which starts to challenge traditional worker–user relationships. It may also mean a focus on personal development as younger workers themselves may be in the process of separating from home: are new services providing a half-way house for them as well?

To date, normalisation training (see Lindley and Wainwright, this volume) has dealt with the oppression of people with disabilities at a historical level and not through experiential approaches which invite workers to acknowledge their own ambivalence towards the people for whom they care. There seems to be a fear that to own such feelings will lead people once again to act out the rejection of disabled people, and a strong peer group culture has grown up which censors such negative feelings and promises a rosy future. Workers need to face the present, and people with disabilities need advocates who have a firm grounding in what is happening. Training and supervision have three functions (see Brown and Ferns 1990): to set the direction for services, to help workers to develop the skills to operate in new ways and to establish a learning culture in which they feel confident enough to learn from experience and monitor their effectiveness.

Focusing on any one element to the exclusion of the others leads to staff feeling disillusioned, incompetent or unrecognised.

Because institutionalised working practices evolved to contain workers' anxieties, any restructuring of working practice has the potential to cause feelings of severe dislocation for staff. This will be especially true if workers are not involved in planning the changes or are not adequately informed of what is happening. The management of change requires that direct care staff, who, as Braisby *et al.* (1988) point out, will play the biggest role in implementing a new philosophy, be meaningfully involved in planning at all levels. Users are also subject to the same anxiety around change; they too need to be involved in planning new services. Failure to do so may result in entrenched resistance to change, born out of un-addressed anxiety and insufficient acknowledgement of the implications for individual workers, many of whom have spent their entire careers in the institution, or users, for whom the institution is home.

Indeed, attention is rarely paid to the rites of passage of leaving an institution, users and staff need to be helped to mourn the loss of friends, status, places and patterns of living. By splitting off the institution from community life, workers forget that institutions were communities of sorts, with all their limitations, and that people with disabilities had real roots which could not be severed without feelings of loss and distress. Ramon (1988) notes that while sociologists have well documented the 'degradation ceremonies' of becoming a psychiatric patient (Garfinkel 1956; Goffman 1961), the issue of leaving the hospital as a life event goes largely un-recognised, despite the body of work charting the importance of dealing with such major life events (Brown and Harris 1978). Failure to acknow-ledge the significance of the event can lead to depression and difficulty in adjustment to new circumstances for both users and staff.

CONCLUSION

In maintaining a 'collective, social defence system', notes Menzies (1970), job satisfaction is decreased as nurses are prevented from caring for the 'whole' person; the prevailing work ethos makes it difficult to cope with patients who will not recover; good work is taken for granted and little praise given; there is little acknowledgement of individuals' contributions and a general disregard of workers' needs. Users receive a service which is also unresponsive to their needs and they may have to live in a persecutory and repressive regime. However, despite these glaring imperfections, insti-tutions did function to manage the hostility of the community towards people who are perceived to be threateningly different and, for the workers, to contain the anxiety inherent in the task of caring. It is largely because of the unconscious nature of these mechanisms that they have become maladaptive through use.

Thus, the organisational structure of the hospital assists staff in doing their job and its removal will inevitably cause anxiety about the autonomy, responsibility and uncertainty of new roles. Lack of consideration of these factors will lead to superficial changes which cause minimal disruption to social defences, but also few real improvements in working practices. The result will be mini-institutions in the community – an outcome which is neither morally fair nor effective for people with disabilities. Training in normalisation will help staff gain insight into the ways and the reasons why people with disabilities are oppressed; however, insight does not mean that such oppression will automatically be reversed. Normalisation presents an opportunity to redress this situation but only if the psychological functions of coping with the anxiety of the work are made conscious and adequately contained through proper training, supervision and attention to the organisation of the work. New services must recognize that the success and viability of any social 'institution' are intimately connected with the structures used to contain anxiety. Understanding these is essential if we are to facilitate real and lasting change in the services people receive.

REFERENCES

Abberley, P. (1987) 'The concept of oppression and the development of a social theory of disability', *Disability Handicap and Society* 2, 1.

Allderidge, P. (1979) 'Hospitals, madhouses and asylums: Cycles in the care of the insane', *British Journal of Psychiatry* 134: 321–34.

Braisby, D., Echlin, R., Hill, S., and Smith, H. (1988) *Changing Futures: Housing and support services for people discharged from psychiatric hospitals*, London: King Edwards Hospital Fund for London.

Brost, M., and Johnson, T. (1982) *Getting to Know You: One approach to service assessment and planning for individuals with disabilities*, Madison: Wisconsin Council on Development Disabilities.

Brown, G., and Harris, T. (1978) *Social Origins of Depression*, London: Tavistock.

Brown, H. (1987) 'Working with parents', in A. Craft (ed.) *Mental Handicap and Sexuality*, Tunbridge Wells: Costello.

Brown, H., and Ferns, P. (1990) *Supervising Staff: Video assisted training pack in the 'Bringing People Back Home' series*, Bexhill: SETRHA.

Finch, J., and Groves, D. (eds) (1983) *A Labour of Love: Women, work and caring*, London: Routledge and Kegan Paul.

Freud, S. (1901) *The Psychopathology of Everyday Life*, Standard Edition, 6, London: Hogarth Press.

Garfinkel, H. (1956) 'Ceremonies of degradation', *American Journal of Sociology*.

Goffman, E. (1961) *Asylums*, Harmondsworth: Penguin.

Kingsley, S., and Smith, H. (1989) *Values for Change: Principles and approaches in designing a local training strategy*, London: King Edwards Hospital Fund for London.

Klein, M. (1937) *Love, Guilt and Reparation*, London: Hogarth Press.

Klein, M. (1940) 'Mourning and its relation to manic-depressive states', *International Journal of Psycho-Analysis*, 21.

Lamb, R. (1979) 'Staff burnout in work with long term patients', *Hospital and Community Psychiatry* 30: 6.

Menzies, I. (1970) *The Functioning of Social Systems as a Defence against Anxiety*, London: Tavistock.

Millar, A. (1987) *For Your Own Good: The roots of violence in child rearing*, London: Virago Press.

Morris, P. (1969) *Put Away: A sociological study of institutions for the mentally retarded*, London: Routledge and Kegan Paul.

O'Brien, J. (1980) 'The principle of normalisation: A foundation for effective services', in J. Gardner, L. Long, R. Nichols, and D. Iagulli (eds) *Program Issues in Developmental Disabilities: A resource manual for surveyors and reviewers*, Baltimore: Paul H. Brookes.

Oswin, M. (1984) *They Keep Going Away: A critical study of short-term residential care services for children who are mentally handicapped*, London: King's Fund.

Parker, G. (1985) *With Due Care and Attention: A review of research on informal care*, Family Policy Studies Centre, Occasional Paper 2.

Ramon, S. (1988) 'Rites of passage upon leaving the psychiatric hospital: Beginning with the user's perspective', unpublished Paper.

Ryan, J. with Thomas, F. (1980) *The Politics of Mental Handicap*, Harmondsworth: Penguin.

Sinason, V. (1986) 'Secondary mental handicap and its relationship to trauma', *Psychoanalytic Psychotherapy* 2, 2: 131–54.

Wolfensberger, W. (1975) *The Origin and Nature of our Institutional Models*, Syracuse: Human Policy Press.

Wolfensberger, W. (1983) *PASSING Normalization Criteria and Ratings Manual* (2nd Edition), Canadian National Institute on Mental Retardation.

Wolfensberger, W. (1987) 'How to Function with Personal Moral Coherency in a Disfunctional (Human Service) World', Workshop offered by the Training Institute for Human Service Planning and Change Agentry, Syracuse University, New York.

7 Social welfare ideologies and normalisation
Links and conflicts

Gillian Dalley

This chapter aims to discuss the concept of normalisation and its relationship to different social welfare ideologies. In so doing, it will be Wolfensberger's (1972) definition of the concept that will be used, as it is this one which most explicitly claims to have an ideological foundation. Other interpretations – notably the early Scandinavian formulation and its current exposition in the United Kingdom – have tended to eschew any claims to theoretical or ideological status. As Emerson describes elsewhere in this volume, the approach currently advocated by O'Brien (O'Brien and Tyne 1981) and the King's Fund 'An Ordinary Life' programme (Towell 1988) concentrates on developing and outlining practical strategies for setting up services which actively promote the concept of normalisation in terms of individual choice, active participation, the development of individual competence and the appropriate location of services. It is Wolfensberger who, in Emerson's terms, does the 'grand theorising'. Thus it is his interpretation that will be examined here for its ideological content.

In looking at Wolfensberger's theorising, this chapter draws attention to some of the implications of his argument. In particular it stresses the major elements of conservatism and moral authoritarianism inherent in his views and goes on to suggest that these may have the effect of reinforcing aspects of the status quo he wishes to overturn. In addition, it argues that alternative ideological approaches may be more successful in achieving some of the objectives claimed for normalisation theory – namely, those of improving the social and moral position of people generally devalued by society at large because of their so-called 'deviant' characteristics. A collectivist approach which stresses the values of mutual support, co-operation and equality of status for all citizens is more likely to nurture devalued people than the individualist tendencies of Wolfensberger's normalisation.

This chapter first examines the ideological content of the theory, demonstrating its conservative character and seeks to set it in a broader context – looking at other, competing, ideological positions. In particular, it compares its relationship to collectivism on the one hand and individualism on the other and looks at how, in practice, a collectivist approach may achieve the objectives that Wolfensberger would claim for normalisation.

IDEOLOGICAL ELEMENTS IN NORMALISATION THEORY

In first setting out the principle of normalisation, Wolfensberger (1972) stressed the importance of the role of ideology in the way human service organisations are structured. He sees services as operating at both a conscious and unconscious level, conditioning the way society and its professional agents think and behave. To reiterate briefly Emerson (this volume), Wolfensberger describes the dynamics underlying society's attitudes to devalued groups through the process of labelling; that is, people are devalued because they are labelled as deviant. To be categorised as deviant may mean that such individuals are seen variably as menaces, subhuman, childlike, diseased, ridiculous. Avoidance reaction to them by society may, at worst, lead to their destruction or, more likely, their segregation from the rest of society. Normalisation, however, contains an ideological imperative which stresses the need to reverse this process of social devaluing.

It is in examining this process of normalisation that we can begin to uncover some of the ideological propositions contained within it. In 1972, Wolfensberger defined normalisation as the 'utilization of means which are as culturally normative as possible, in order to establish and/or maintain personal behaviours and characteristics which are as culturally normative as possible'. Some time later he wrote that 'the most explicit and highest goal of normalisation must be the creation, support and defence of valued social roles for people who are at risk of social devaluation' (1983).

The key phrases in both these extracts are 'as culturally normative as possible' and 'valued social roles'. It is worth noting his concentration on roles rather than persons. His starting point tends to be the roles that people occupy rather than people as the persons they are. In so doing, he is less concerned with the attributes that make people fall into the category of deviant or devalued, than with the roles they then come to possess. Thus he does not discuss the nature of those attributes, for example intellectual or physical impairments, nor does he analyse the relationship between the condition (the sum of those attributes) and the ensuing role. He recognises that historically, impaired, 'retarded' or otherwise devalued people are feared, ridiculed or loathed by society – hence their destruction or segregation. But he does not discuss the notion that if society is to offer them valued roles, then there must be a *fundamental* re-evaluation of those categories of persons *qua* persons. This latter approach is similar to that found in the Scandinavian model of normalisation, which goes some way in addressing this particular issue (Bank-Mikkelsen 1980; Perrin and Nirje 1985).

By failing to address this fundamental aspect of ideology, that is, the way in which impaired individuals are perceived, assessed and esteemed as individuals (or not) by society, Wolfensberger omits an essential first stage in his analysis. He fails to tackle the nature of ideology or to recognise that ideology is not like an overcoat – something to put on or take off or change completely as desired – but something more subtle, more complex and more profound. Fallers (1961) has defined ideology as 'that part of culture which is actively concerned with the establishment and defence of patterns of belief and value'. Changing the ideological base of beliefs and attitudes is not something that can be achieved by exhortation: it is a force which defines and motivates fields of action in a most powerful way – a way which is not changed by whim or mere technique. Wolfensberger, however, seems to suggest that by adopting his training strategies in unproblematic fashion, 'society' through the agency of its 'human service professionals' will alter its perception of devalued people.

Wolfensberger, though, presents us with a contradiction: in spite of his assertion that the principles which he is expounding are a powerful tool for change, over the years he has come to believe that there is a societal conspiracy to destroy devalued groups and that contemporary de-institutionalisation policies are doomed to failure regardless of the original aims of the policies and the motives of those who promulgate them. Thus 'the soul of this society' is

> engaged in a very well-hidden policy of genocidal destruction of certain of its rejected and unwanted classes, especially those who have impairments that render them of little value to others in an increasingly utilitarian value context.
>
> (Wolfensberger 1987: 141)

Whether he believes his own techniques will fare any better in the face of what he perceives as society-wide hostility is unclear. A point that should be stressed, however, is that by focusing on 'role', emphasis is inevitably placed on behaviour and techniques of behavioural adjustment. It is in examining these that some of the ideological elements in normalisation become clearer, notably its conservatism, moral authoritarianism and emphasis on conformity.

CONSERVATISM

While Wolfensberger emphasises that the concept must be culturally specific, 'because cultures vary in their norms' (1987), he fails to acknowledge to any great extent that a given society may not in itself be culturally uniform. It would be a mistake to ignore the fact that societies are made up of disparate groups with their own interests, their own ideologies, their own goals and their own norms. In arguing that norms are culture-specific, Wolfensberger is in danger of assuming that the norms of the dominant group, the dominant ideology, should necessarily become the model focus for normalisation strategies. This would inevitably mean ignoring, for example, the differing norms associated with class, gender and ethnicity, an unfortunate prescription in our modern, multi-cultural and heterogeneous society. It implies an acceptance of the status quo (which is governed by the dominant ideology) and a conservative unwillingness to challenge existing norms.

MORAL AUTHORITARIANISM

The conservative focus on norms, along with the failure to recognise the fact of cultural heterogeneity, leads to a tendency to be prescriptive about what constitutes normative behaviour. The stress on teaching or training 'deviant' clients in forms of behaviour which will not mark them out as deviant seems to imply an acceptance of the original diagnosis of them as 'deviant':

> For instance, the normalization principle demands that a person should be taught not merely to walk, but to walk with a normal gait; that he use normal movements and normal expressive behavior patterns; that he dress like other persons of his age; and that his diet be such as to assure normal weight.
>
> (Wolfensberger 1972: 33)

Yet Wolfensberger says that deviancy is a social role imposed by others, *not* something inherent in the individual's condition. Questions, therefore, have to be asked about the moral justification for such prescriptive demands. Are they likely to improve the quality of the client's life because they are offering alternative ways of behaving which are intrinsically better? (for example, an appropriate diet will ensure good health). Or are such patterns of behaviour being prescribed because they will lessen the hostility of others towards them? (for example, people may not like looking at fat people who are also disabled in some way). The latter may improve the quality of life for the client in a very limited way by diminishing the hostility of outsiders, but it certainly does not tackle the fundamental moral issue of whose interests are being promoted by the prescription of such normative behaviour.

CONFORMITY

The essence, then, of normalisation seems to be conformity; little value is placed on diversity and difference. At its most extreme, the pressure to conform may require radical measures

> Cosmetic surgery can often eliminate or reduce a stigma, and can be as effective in enhancing a person's acceptability as teaching adaptive skills, changing his conduct or working on his feelings.
>
> (Wolfensberger 1972: 34)

The argument seems to be that people are perceived as belonging to devalued groups, therefore let us pretend to the outside world that they do not, by offering them techniques of behaviour or other adaptive measures, so that they will no longer be marked out as members of those devalued groups:

> Since deviancy is, by definition, in the eyes of the beholder, it is only realistic to attend not only to the limitations in a person's repertoire of potential behaviour but to attend as much or even more to those characteristics and behaviours which mark a person as deviant in the sight of others. For instance, wearing a hearing aid may be a greater obstacle to finding and keeping a job than being hard of hearing.
>
> (Wolfensberger 1972: 28)

This does little to challenge fundamental attitudes held by society at large towards disability. Further, the consequences are great for those who *cannot* conform and who remain visibly, through physical or behavioural impairment, members of those devalued groups. They will form a residual, devalued population, forever stigmatised.

Wolfensberger does, in fairness, recognise that society's views must be challenged and changed:

> We should work for greater acceptance of differentness of modes of grooming, dressing, speaking; of skin color, race, religious and national origin; of appearance, age, sex, intelligence, and education. Also encouraged should be greater acceptance of the physically and sensory handicapped, the epileptic, the emotionally disordered, and perhaps the sexually unorthodox.
>
> (Wolfensberger 1972: 41)

Requiring devalued individuals to change *their* behaviour so that it conforms to what is regarded as 'normal' will not achieve the fundamental re-evaluation of dominant ideological attitudes that is necessary (see also Brown and Smith, this volume).

COMPETING SOCIAL WELFARE IDEOLOGIES

Normalisation is not, of course, the only moral framework for tackling issues of oppression and disadvantage. It has been argued elsewhere (Dalley 1988) that modern social welfare policies have been characterised by a pull between two contrasting ideologies – notably, possessive individualism and collectivism. It is worth examining these two ideologies in more detail as they provide a useful framework for understanding the ideological imperatives that direct normalisation. Since the inception of the welfare state and before, there has been a tradition of the state developing social provision for the poor and the dependent. During this century, we have seen the introduction of state pensions for retired people, income maintenance for the unemployed, the National Health Service providing health care free at the point of use for all, a variety of social services and a number of financial benefits for the sick and disabled. The welfare state (in spite of some demonstrable failings) has been celebrated as an exemplary expression of collectivist values made real.

In earlier centuries, too, there have been expressions of collective support. Surprisingly, Poor Law provision was relatively generous, especially to widows and the elderly (Smith 1984), at least until the New Poor Law 1834 was implemented. This introduced the harsh institutional framework of the workhouse and the principle of 'less eligibility' whereby poor law relief given to the able-bodied pauper should never make his or her condition superior to that of the poorest working labourer. Further, the meagre relief that was provided had to be given within the confines of the workhouse. Thus the division between the deserving and undeserving poor was established. But collective forms of support persisted in other ways: the trades unions and friendly societies provided welfare and financial services for their members and religious institutions frequently took the lead in other forms of welfare provision for the poor and needy. Thus there has been a long tradition of collective expressions of social responsibility in a variety of forms.

However, during this same period, society has also been characterised by its strong emphasis on possessive individualism. Certain sources (Macfarlane 1978) argue that such a philosophy dates back as far as the Middle Ages, at least in England. The extended corporate family, which characterised many peasant societies in Europe and other parts of the world, was never greatly in evidence in this country. The essence of possessive individualism, according to Macpherson (1962), lies in its sense of privacy and freedom from intrusion and in its conception of the individual as proprietor of his/her own person and capacities: 'the human essence is freedom from dependence on the will of others and freedom is the function of possession'.

Lukes (1973) expresses it similarly: 'individualism offers a private existence within a public world, an area within which the individual is or should be left alone by others and able to do and think whatever he [*sic*] chooses'.

The significance of the private, home-centred nuclear family is a central feature of possessive individualism – with man the breadwinner operating in the public domain, supported at home in the private realm by wife and children. It became the ideal model for modern society although, as is now well known, such a model is far from universal in practice. A report by the Study Commission on the Family (1983) (later the Family Policy Studies Centre) shows that in the twenty years between 1961 and 1980 the percentage of families conforming to the ideal 'married couple with children' model fell from 38 per cent to 32 per cent of all household types. Nevertheless, the model of the private, nuclear family has come to underpin many of the principles which inform current social policies – in spite, it can be argued, of the contradiction that this generates. Thus the concept and structure of welfare is based on a concept and structure of collective provision; but a model of possessive individualism constantly intervenes and cuts across it. Collective responsibility for welfare is broadly accepted and valued (West *et al.* 1984) but the models of care widely advocated tend to be those based on the individualistic family model of care.

This is a model which proposes that when care or support is required – and the immediate (nuclear) family cannot provide it – then what is offered by both statutory and non-statutory services should mimic the family model as closely as possible. Institutional and residential care have become unacceptable to policy makers and practitioners not only because empirically they are frequently found wanting, but also because they do not match the model of (surrogate) family care which is deemed to be the only valid form when 'own family' is unavailable. Furthermore, the norms and values of the family model of care match its structural form; privacy, independence, an emphasis on living lives enclosed in small units, dependent on a small, limited range of 'significant others' (surrogate family members). Meanwhile there is an assumption that collective forms of caring for people are both stigmatised and stigmatising.

This is especially important in relation to the emphasis placed on community care policies in the 1980s and, indeed, in relation to the values and strategies espoused by normalisation. Care in the community, the paramountcy of family forms of care, the stress placed on 'own home' regardless, frequently, of the isolation this entails, becomes the ideal to be strived for in all circumstances. Most importantly, the professionals involved in organising and providing care services – in Wolfensberger's terms, the human service professionals – have demonstrated overwhelming support for this approach. It has become the dominant welfare ideology of the day, promoted by a host of interested parties, central government, senior civil servants, professional associations in the health and social services, together with field-level professionals and voluntary organisations.

In the face of this overwhelming support, the client at the receiving end of policy rarely has the opportunity to assent or dissent. Services are already planned, designed and budgeted for by the time the client comes into the picture. Furthermore, professionals often adopt highly judgemental views of those clients or their supporters who adopt contrary views (the old person wishing to go into a nursing home; the parents of a mentally handicapped son or daughter seeking residential care; sons and daughters with elderly parents suffering from dementia trying to place them in residential care). The views of the social welfare establishment prevail.

Yet contrary views are beginning to be expressed. There is mounting evidence (Jones and Poletti 1985; Great Britain Parliament, House of Commons 1985) from many sources – North America, Italy, the United Kingdom – that community care policies are not working (indeed, Wolfensberger (1987) refers to this fact). The reasons which are advanced for this failure vary: some argue that it is due to a failure of will on the part of government; others argue that it is due to lack of resources being put into the community; yet others (Wolfensberger 1987, for example) argue that it is because society is determined to destroy the devalued groups in question, whichever policy is in the ascendant. It may be that disillusionment with the policies will signal a reassertion of collectivist attitudes. Alternatives to the private, inward-looking family model of care in the form of group care may, after all, be worth preserving. Whitehead (this volume) traces the development of normalisation and its relationship to the development of other social policies in this country. This historical analysis, though, does not examine the ideological fit between normalisation and the philosophical imperatives behind the development of social welfarism. Are there ideological links between these concepts?

NORMALISATION AND COLLECTIVISM

Deeply embedded in the ideology of collectivism are the principles of equity and egalitarianism: collectivists would argue that it is the duty of society to provide support for all citizens according to their need, especially in times of want, sickness or dependency. Citizens should have equal rights of access to such support regardless of attributes such as class, gender, race, (dis)ability and the like. The basis for that support is one of fellowship (Meacher 1982), incorporating the values of sharing, altruism and co-operation. Similarly, one of the chief motivations underpinning the concept of normalisation has been the concern to enable members of devalued groups to participate fully and on valued terms in the life of the community. Their rights to the support and benefits conferred by society are the same as those of any other citizens. Thus the twin notions of the valued status of all citizens and of equality of access – be it to the full life of the community or to the nurturing and protective support of the collectivity – are common to the philosophies of both collectivism and normalisation. On these terms, they have much in common.

But in other respects there are some important differences. Although propounders of individualism argue that collectivists do not respect individual freedom sufficiently, that is, they subordinate the interests of the individual to those of the mass, collectivists would argue that this is not so: they value individual freedom as long as it does not impinge on or deny the freedom of other individuals. They might, under these circumstances, find the prescriptive elements inherent in some of the practice of normalisation unacceptable, seeing them as an erosion or denial of clients' rights. Care for dependent people, according to the collectivist view, ought to uphold a number of principles designed to broaden the range of opportunities for people requiring care and to reduce their dependence on privatised, family-based care. These should include the ability for the dependent person to be responsible for his or her own life choices; the capacity of the care system to be responsive to individual needs and choices (of both the cared for and the carer); the opportunity to develop wide and varied personal relationships; economic security; and the acceptance by the wider community of responsibility for care.

These latter goals are undoubtedly analogous to those espoused by normalisation; however, the translation of these goals into practice divides the two concepts. In practice, collectivism means that the provision of care does not depend on the altruistic self-sacrifice of individual carers or the consignment of dependent people to the warehouses of institutional care, but instead should be based on the principles of group concern, shared care and mutual support. Collective settings, as opposed to institutional settings, may foster these principles more easily than care provided in a fragmented way in individual, often isolated, homes. Such settings, based on mutual support and respect for all members (be they able-bodied or dependent), actively value diversity and difference. They might involve groups of individuals living together under the same roof, with some in need of care or support and others providing it, but all participating in an active, integrated communal life (while at the same time having relationships where desired with others outside the group). Such living arrangements have prevailed in different times and in different cultures and have been highly valued by those involved in them (Dalley 1988).

This represents a clear split with normalisation which requires members of devalued groups to move towards the prevailing norms of small group living. It would seem that the fundamental difference between collectivism and normalisation lies in the belief that living collectively is either life-enhancing or inevitably leads to stigma and devaluation.

NORMALISATION AND INDIVIDUALISM

It has been noted earlier that there has been a continuing struggle during the history of welfare provision between the ideologies of collectivism and possessive individualism. Many would argue that in spite of the establishment of the welfare state in the 1940s, the dominant ideology has been one of individualism, particularly during the 1980s (Bean *et al.* 1985). Thus, there is an emphasis placed on privacy, independence, the separation of public and private domains, an acceptance of accompanying notions of gender division and women's subordination and the preaching of a creed of sturdy self-reliance. Providing collective support has been relabelled the 'dependency culture', mutual inter-dependency is deprecated. Individuals are expected to provide care and support for themselves and their families and where this is not possible, surrogate forms of family care are advocated, while other possibilities are denied or under-funded (Dalley 1988).

Again, there is an ambiguous match with normalisation. Wolfensberger stresses that normalisation is a 'culture-specific' concept. Not only is it culture-specific, but in practice it supports the status quo and the dominant individualised ideology of care. An ideology that advocates self-reliance, traditional gendered roles and private solutions to issues of social responsibility may be inimical to the capacity of individuals for development. Yet the creed of privacy, independence and family care is one to which normalisation strongly adheres.

CONCLUSION

Drawing out the links and defining the contrasts between normalisation and current social welfare ideologies is a perplexing task. On the one hand Wolfensberger (1972) clearly states that normalisation is an ideological construct; on the other, he says that 'the normalization principle can be viewed as being neutral as to whether a specific deviant person or group *should be* normalized. That decision must be based on criteria and values which exist independent of the normalization principle' (ibid.).

Wolfensberger is therefore claiming for normalisation the status of both a moral system *and* a morally neutral technique. Thus he acknowledges the strong ideological component within normalisation which relates to the struggle to secure full rights for members of devalued groups to become actively participating citizens. In this, it has much in common with the principles underlying the collectivist conception of welfare and social responsibility. However, the emphasis on changing people, through modification of behaviour, appearance and attitudes rather than focusing on the paramount need to change society's attitudes towards disability, runs counter to the egalitarian principle of valuing individuals for themselves whatever the nature of their (dis)ability. Even if we accept that normalisation is a morally neutral technique, it is a technique which has undoubted ideological consequences. Because it tends to support the status quo in the United Kingdom, it is supporting an individualistic ideology which favours family-based or family-surrogate models of care and emphasises individual competence and self-reliance. This chapter has argued that such an ideology is intrinsically damaging to many of the people on whose behalf normalisation is being advocated.

The concept of normalisation, then, is complex and in some senses contradictory. It has elements which have something in common with the two major – and competing – social welfare ideologies prevailing in Britain today, but it has other traits to which neither of those ideologies would subscribe. When it is more modestly presented as a means for demanding full and equal citizenship for all those who would otherwise remain devalued, it is both more coherent and more morally acceptable.

REFERENCES

Bank-Mikkelsen, N. (1980) 'Denmark', in R.J. Flynn and K.E. Nitsch (eds) *Normalisation, Social Integration and Community Services*, Austin, Texas: Pro-Ed.

Bean, P., Ferris, J., and Whynes, D. (eds) (1985) *In Defence of Welfare*, London: Tavistock.

Dalley, G. (1988) *Ideologies of Caring: Rethinking community and collectivism*, London: Macmillan.

Fallers, L.A. (1961) 'Ideology and culture in Uganda nationalism', *American Anthropologist* 63, 19.

Great Britain Parliament, House of Commons (1985) 'Community care, with special reference to adult mentally ill and mentally handicapped people', Second report from the Social Services Select Committee, session 1984–85, London: HMSO.

Jones, K., and Poletti, A. (1985) 'Understanding the Italian experience', *British Journal of Psychiatry* 146.

Lukes, S. (1973) *Individualism*, Oxford: Basil Blackwell.

Macfarlane, A. (1978) *The Origins of English Individualism*, Oxford: Basil Blackwell.

Macpherson, C.B. (1962) *The Political Theory of Possessive Individualism*, Oxford: Oxford University Press.

Meacher, M. (1982) *Socialism with a Human Face*, London: George Allen and Unwin.

O'Brien, J., and Tyne, A. (1981) *The Principle of Normalisation: A foundation for effective services*, London: Campaign for Mentally Handicapped People.

Perrin, B., and Nirje, B. (1985) 'Setting the record straight: A critique of some frequent misconceptions of the normalisation principle', *Australian and New Zealand Journal of Developmental Disabilities* 11.

Smith, J.E. (1984) 'Widowhood and ageing in traditional English society', *Ageing and Society* 4, 4.

Study Commission on the Family (1983) *Families in the Future: A policy agenda for the '80s*, London: Study Commission on the Family.

Towell, D. (1988) *An Ordinary Life in Practice*, London: King's Fund Centre.

West, P., Illsley, R., and Kelman, H. (1984) 'Public preferences for the care of dependency groups', *Social Science and Medicine* 18, 4.

Wolfensberger, W. (1972) *The Principle of Normalization in Human Services*, Toronto: National Institute on Mental Retardation.

Wolfensberger, W. (1983) 'Social role valorization: A proposed new term for the principle of normalization', *Mental Retardation* 21, 6.

Wolfensberger, W. (1987) 'Values in the funding of social services', *American Journal of Mental Deficiency* 92, 2.

8   The limits to integration?

Sue Szivos

This chapter unpacks some of the assumptions contained within normalisation about integration. It is written from the position of a psychologist
concerned about some of the basic psychological processes that advocates
of normalisation have overlooked. Although many examples will be drawn
from the area of learning difficulties, examples will also be taken from
other groups, highlighting the relevance of this critique to all people to
whom the theory of normalisation has been applied.

The chapter will start by examining two 'classic' formulations of normalisation (Wolfensberger's and Nirje's) and the different basic assumptions each makes about 'difference' and physical and social integration. It
will conclude by asking questions about creating a group identity based on
solidarity rather than dispersal. Such a philosophy could be described, by
analogy, with feminism and post-feminism, as 'post-normalisation'. I want,
however, to make it clear that post-normalisation does not mean returning
to the ghettoisation of the institutional era, but moving to a climate in which
account can be taken of people's needs and desires for affiliation.

COMPETING DEFINITIONS OF NORMALISATION

Wolfensberger's definition of normalisation is by now so well known that
it barely requires to be repeated. However, since a primary aim of this
chapter is to examine some of the different assumptions made by Wolfensberger and Nirje, it is reprinted here that normalisation is the

> utilization of means which are as culturally normative as possible in
> order to establish and/or maintain personal behaviours which are as
> culturally normative as possible.
>
> (Wolfensberger 1972: 28)

As this definition implies, normalisation focuses on the two dimensions of
'means' and 'behaviours' as the way of breaking the vicious circle of

negative behaviour, imagery and ill-treatment of devalued people. The latter dimension refers to

> Eliciting, shaping and maintaining normative skills and habits in persons by means of direct physical and social interaction with them . . . by working indirectly through . . . social systems such as family, classroom, school, work setting . . . government.
>
> (ibid.: 32)

This means maximising the person's behavioural competence beyond the point of being merely physically adaptive, to the point of being socially normative:

> The interaction ['behaviour'] dimension . . . implies that we teach a person to exercise those behaviours which elicit [positive] social judgement [gait; weight control; dress; expressive behaviour patterns] even if they have little practical problem-solving value.
>
> (ibid.: 33)

The interpretation dimension ['means'] is more concerned with public attitudes. It involves

> Presenting, managing, addressing, labelling and interpreting individual persons in a manner emphasizing their similarities to rather than differences from others; shaping, presenting and interpreting . . . social systems . . . so that the persons in them are perceived as culturally normative as possible; shaping cultural values, attitudes and stereotypes so as to elicit maximal feasible cultural acceptance of differences.
>
> (ibid.: 32)

This also extends to using ordinary buildings and other life spaces, such as work environments; these should be small, dispersed, and in the usual residential, work and leisure areas.

Wolfensberger, therefore, advocates ending the use of derogatory and belittling labelling and demeaning environments, and minimising what he calls 'deviancy juxtaposition', that is, grouping deviant clients with other deviant clients or devalued groups. This not only minimises the total perceived deviance, but also provides more suitable role models for non-deviant behaviour (bringing together the 'means' and 'behaviour' dimensions), preventing the formation of a 'subculture of deviance':

> When deviant individuals work for and with other deviant persons, and when deviant persons socialize intensively and perhaps exclusively with each other, it is almost inevitable that a climate or subculture of deviancy is created which exacerbates rather than reverses the deviancy of those

within this climate or subculture. Finally, at a given time, a person generally has the potential of forming a limited number of social ties and relationships. Usually, he will fill his 'friendship vacancies' with people he encounters in the social systems close to him. The likelihood of filling one's relationship needs is in direct proportion to the percentage of such persons in one's social systems . . . the perceived deviance of both groups is likely to increase, and even their adaptive behaviour often decreases. Far from being habilitative, the chances of habilitation for . . . the . . . client group is likely to be reduced by such measures.

(ibid.: 36)

In 1983, Wolfensberger renamed normalisation 'social role valorisation'. This followed considerable criticism centred around the concept of normality: the meanings of the word 'normal' are confusing and problematic; what is statistically normative is not necessarily the best; the words 'normal' and 'deviant' are heavily value-laden and Wolfensberger did not always use them in the neutral sense he claimed (witness the above passage). The major shift of emphasis in social role valorisation was the change in meaning of the term normal/normative meaning 'statistically normative' to meaning 'socially valued' (Wolfensberger 1984). In social role valorisation, the 'means' and 'behaviour' dimensions are renamed 'image enhancement' and 'competency enhancement' but the strategies for service providers remain essentially the same, as does their major aim which is 'to create or support socially valued roles for people in society' (1980: 23; cf. 1983: 234).

While Wolfensberger's definition has as its focus the normative images, competencies and behaviours demanded of people and their services, in contrast, Nirje's emphasis is on making available to people with mental handicaps normative patterns and conditions of everyday life (Nirje 1969) and on the individual's subjective experience of self. A normal environment or rhythm of life

provides the handicapped adult with the range of conditions and experiences of life that will support his self confidence and feelings of adulthood . . . trainees have to acquire self confidence by experiencing themselves as capable of passing over various thresholds of challenge and growth.

(Nirje 1972: 181)

With a lessened emphasis on external images and behaviour, Nirje has a rather different set of assumptions about the way 'difference' is perceived. First, there is less focus on bringing the individual's behaviour up to some culturally acceptable norm; and second, because 'difference' is more acceptable in itself, group activities can be viewed much more positively:

In society, one common and accepted way to assert oneself and the endeavours one feels identified with is through co-operation within social bodies of common interests and goals . . . Through these bodies, common feelings and needs can be shared and expressed, and common demands formulated . . . Overt and collective expression of thoughts and feelings is not only a traditional therapeutic device to relieve tension, but it is also the way of cultural exchange and politics. It provides a medium of identification with one's self, helps define a 'cause' and serves as a medium for establishing meaningful and functional social relationships.

(Nirje 1972: 177)

Such groups can provide an opportunity for social interaction and self expression which may otherwise not be available in the same quantity or quality. For instance, it may be that some handicapped young adults will find it easier to mix with the non-handicapped but that [others] will have much greater difficulties in meeting their needs in an integrated fashion. Many may wish to join a self-directed group in order to state this hunger.

(Nirje 1972: 186)

There are several reasons why Wolfensberger's formulation rather than Nirje's has been taken up by British and American services. Most obviously, Wolfensberger was writing specifically 'for the purposes of a North American audience' (1972: 28). His work on Program Analysis of Service Systems (PASS) (Wolfensberger and Thomas 1983) provided a systematic blueprint for evaluating services; and his scientific language (Nirje's language in contrast has been called 'pre-scientific and intuitive' – Briton 1979) gave his writings an empiricist persuasiveness and set mental handicap in the context of fashionable theories of deviance. However, these merits have been the source of criticism. Briton (1979) notes that

. . . almost completely absent from Wolfensberger's discourse is a vocabulary that Nirje draws on constantly – a vocabulary of persons, applying to human subjectivity and allowing us to talk of the retarded person's experience of self and its internally measured quality. What replaces it is a vocabulary which applies to human beings only through an external view of individuated behaviours and their applicability.

(Briton 1979: 227–8)

Yet as Briton continues, without subjective benefits, normalisation becomes no more than 'a blind endorsement of conformity'.

It is also necessary to question Wolfensberger's 'instrumentalist reasoning' (Briton 1979) which sees the dispersal of people with disabilities throughout the community as a prerequisite for reduced visibility, appropriate role models and increasingly appropriate behaviour. In general terms, few would disagree that complex social and psychological processes ensure that much abnormal behaviour is generated by abnormal situations. This may be due both to the internalisation by the individual of low and distorted expectations as well as the limited opportunities afforded to him or her. Conversely, treating people with kindness and respect leads to enhanced action and the internalisation of self-respect which in turn promote positive behaviour and interactions. However, many of the assumptions about role modelling and social acceptance have not been substantiated. Indeed, the very concepts of roles and socially created deviance may be outdated and seriously inadequate to describe the dynamics underlying social responses to people with disabilities.

Therefore, without wishing to decry the enormous steps taken in bringing to public attention the appalling conditions inflicted on individuals in large custodial settings, this chapter will seek to examine some assumptions about social integration and the psychological processes involved which are inadequately addressed by Wolfensberger's perspective.

NORMALISATION AND SOCIAL POLICY: A CASE OF PERSUASIVE DEFINITION?

Many words have two kinds of meaning: descriptive (denotation) and emotive (connotation). Stevenson (1944) points out that propagandists and moralists have this in common: that they make use of the strong emotive force imbued in certain terms in order to gain acceptance of ideas that they subsume under those terms. He calls this 'persuasive definition':

> ... a great many definitions of emotive terms are persuasive, in intent and effect. Our language abounds with words which, like culture, have both a vague descriptive meaning and a rich emotive meaning. The descriptive meaning of them all is subject to constant redefinition. The words are prizes which each man seeks to bestow upon the qualities of his own choice.
>
> (Stevenson 1944: 212)

To pursue Stevenson's argument into the area of human services, many words like 'normal', 'community', 'deviant' and 'institution' have emotive connotations which are highly persuasive when it comes to forming recommendations for social policy. Lippman (1977) says of 'potentially valuable words ... [like] normalization, deinstitutionalisation, and mainstreaming,

> It may be that they are already functioning as flaglike symbols, calling for the automatic salute rather than the thoughtful consideration that could lead to meaningful social change for retarded individuals.
>
> (1977: 301)

As the definitions of normalisation cited earlier demonstrate, 'normal' and 'normalisation' mean quite different things to Nirje and Wolfensberger. A similar case could be made for the twin concepts of institution/deinstitutionalisation. Since Goffman (1982) and before (for example, Abel and Kinder 1942) the term 'institution' has come to stand for dehumanising practices, segregation and the mortification of the personality, a far cry from the educative and humanitarian impulses which motivated Seguin and other reformers responsible for their inception. In the same year that the DHSS circular Better Services for the Mentally Handicapped (1971) appeared, committed to the principle that people should not be unnecessarily segregated and that the hospital population should be halved by 1991, President Nixon's government coined the term 'de-institutionalisation' to characterise the goal of reducing by a third the number of people living in state institutions (Lippman 1977).

The danger with persuasive definition lies, of course, in assuming that any practices bearing the emotionally positive label are necessarily 'good'. In fact, a quantity of evidence testifies that merely discharging people from institutions does not necessarily alleviate human suffering and that smaller residential services may perpetuate institutional models of care (Balla 1976; Baroff 1981; Landesman-Dwyer *et al.* 1980; Scheerenberger 1974; Tyne 1978). Bercovici (1981) describes some reasons why this may be the case: the need to maintain professional distance; the need for devalued staff to devalue others. In short, small size may be a necessary condition for humanitarian care, but it is certainly not a sufficient one.

A similar danger is discernible in the use of the term 'community', a concept which has entered the arena of social policy as a highly desirable alternative to institutional care. In 1963, President John Kennedy affirmed the nation's responsibility to provide care in the community to its mentally ill and mentally retarded members. In 1975, the director of the National Institute of Mental Health advocated the release 'to the community' of all institutionalised patients who have been given 'adequate preparation for such a change' (Archer and Gruenberg 1982). Similarly, in Britain, the Jay report (1979) recommended the transfer of care of people with learning difficulties from the hospital and health services to the community and social services.

Yet as many writers (Abraham 1989; Clarke 1982; McNamara 1978; Scheerenberger 1974; Thomas 1983) have pointed out, 'community' is a term which fulfils the requirements of vagueness necessary for persuasive definition in having at least two meanings: a socio-political-geographical area and a friendship network. The danger lies in confusing the two meanings in a glow of nostalgia and fantasy so that the geographical location is expected to yield friendship networks. In fact, with a few noteworthy exceptions, individuals in today's society tend not to draw upon their geographical community for social support (that is, friendships) but rather rely upon the sophisticated use of travel and communications technology to maintain extended friendship and kinship networks. As Clarke puts it,

> The accessibility to any individual of various resources may depend on the structure and size of his personal network and on the nature of the interpersonal linkages that make up the network. The resources involved may be tangible ones, such as information about jobs or homes, or intangibles, such as sociability or emotional support.
>
> (Clarke 1982: 460)

While the Jay report (1979) went some way towards spelling out what community care would entail, in particular at least a doubling of staff, the use of the word 'community' has not always been followed through with appropriate attention to the responsibilities involved. Archer and Gruenberg (1982) were 'impressed by the ambiguities in [the] definition of community alternatives'. According to them,

> The 'deinstitutionalisation' policies leading to the dramatic reductions in state mental hospital census transferred financial responsibility for the chronically mentally ill patient from state Mental Health Departments to the Social Welfare systems. A crisis of patient neglect has arisen because no similar transfer of responsibility for their care and treatment has taken place.
>
> (Archer and Gruenberg 1982: 458)

We must ask ourselves whether the similar disagreement between what constitutes health care and social care that is the legacy of the 1990 NHS and Community Care Act, may not contribute to similar crises of care in this country. We already have evidence that a shortfall between rhetoric and responsibility exists. Ryan and Thomas (1980) demonstrate that although hospital places in Britain for children with mental handicaps decreased from 6,648 in 1970 to 4,263 in 1976, local authority residential places remained the same as in 1969, and the proportion of NHS capital spent on mental handicap services dropped between 1970 and 1975, despite commitments to make them a priority. The Audit Commission (1986) similarly pointed to the slow progress of community care in not always keeping pace with the run-down of NHS long-stay institutions: for people with mental health problems in 1986, there were 25,000 fewer beds than ten years ago, but only 9,000 more day places, and '. . . no one knows what happens to many people after they are discharged'. This report also pointed out the uneven pattern of service provision: receiving services depends as much on where one lives as on what one needs.

These figures imply that many people who would formerly have been the responsibility of health authorities are now being cared for at home; as Braddock (1981) demonstrates, this is not surprising given that this is the cheaper option. It therefore becomes pertinent to ask how many informal carers are being, and will continue to be, exploited by community care? Caring for people with disabilities can be demanding and stressful, but at least at the end of their shift, paid staff can shut the door and go home. Yet many family members and friends experience intolerable stress (cf. Pahl and Quine 1987) because of policies which have a hidden agenda of cutting costs. Furthermore, community care runs a high risk of overt sexism in exploiting the more developed sense of social responsibility of women carers (see Brown and Smith, this volume). Nor does the exploitation stop at informal carers: Mansell *et al.* (1987) and Allen *et al.* (1988) note that most formal carers are young unmarried women because the wages are too low to attract people with family and other financial responsibilities and commitments. Staff also regularly work more than three hours per week unpaid overtime, just to keep services functioning at base level.

This section has examined the risk that propagandists and moralists alike may use persuasive definition to push through policies which may have hidden agendas and inadequate funding and whose appeal rests at least partly on the emotive terms in which they are couched. Enough is known about institutions at their worst to make a homily against community care abhorrent (Ryan and Thomas 1980), but it is important to be wary of the pursuit of flagwords without due attention to the social and psychological assumptions they embody.

MISGUIDED MAINSTREAMING?

Mainstreaming, the American interpretation of the 'least restrictive alternative' in education, and the term for what is more usually referred to in Britain as integrated education, entered the American legislative framework with the Education for all Handicapped Children Act (1975), which stated:

> To the maximum extent appropriate, handicapped children . . . are educated with children who are not handicapped . . . and special class, separate schooling or other removal of handicapped children from the regular educational environment occurs only when the nature or severity of the handicap is such that education in regular classes . . . cannot be achieved satisfactorily.
>
> (PL 94–142)

The principle of integrated education received British parliamentary support with the Education Act (1981) which affirmed the responsibility of the mainstream school environment to meet, as far as possible, the special needs of children with learning difficulties. However, Gresham (1982) defined how mainstreaming is based on three faulty assumptions: first, that mainstreamed placements would increase the number of social interactions between disabled and non-disabled children; second, that such placements would increase the social acceptance of disabled children; and third, that disabled children would model the behaviours of non-disabled children because of increased exposure to them. For Gresham, mainstreaming is misguided because: disabled children do not necessarily have the requisite social skills to elicit peer acceptance; these skills are not taught; and increased social isolation and a more restrictive environment are a likely consequence unless provision for social skills training can be made.

It becomes necessary therefore, to question Wolfensberger's assumptions about the propensity of people with disabilities to model whatever behaviour they see around them, whether 'abnormal' or 'normal'. This is not to deny that modelling is a powerful learning strategy, nor that the role models to whom people are exposed are important. However, any evidence for such modelling tends to be anecdotal, and could be explained in other ways. For example, the deviant behaviour witnessed in mental handicap hospitals could be a result of reduced opportunities to behave otherwise, or of impoverished interpersonal interactions. It has also been noted that people with learning difficulties find it more difficult to benefit from 'incidental' (that is, unstructured) learning than do non-handicapped people. But this is the kind of learning which is involved when modelling one's behaviour on someone else (as advocated by Wolfensberger). Moreover, if skills training is undertaken, the lessons learned may not be transferred to new social situations (Gresham 1985). This means that while it is undoubtedly important for disabled and non-disabled people to experience each other's company, the success of such experiences is not guaranteed, and considerable support may be necessary (cf. McConkey *et al.* 1983a and b).

A further assumption about the dispersal of people in the community is that it reduces the visibility of their disabilities. Again, while in broad terms it is undoubtedly true that a large group of people who are identifiably different will be more visible than a smaller group, it does not follow that the optimum size for social interaction is as low as one or two. Szivos (1989) found that some Further Education students experienced anxiety when joining unsupervised mainstream activities such as using the college canteen, and one young woman reported joining her younger sister's class at lunchtimes to avoid being harassed by her own non-handicapped classmates. Gilkey and Zetlin (1987) observed some handicapped young adults in a variety of settings with non-handicapped peers. They found that the handicapped young people took part in very few interactions. Gilkey and

Zetlin explain this by noting that the special students were very aware of their status as 'retarded' or 'outcasts', and may have avoided social interaction with non-handicapped peers in order to avoid rejection. Moreover, their teacher's behaviour, in encouraging the students to mingle among their non-handicapped peers so as to prevent their being so noticeable, actually prevented them from forming friendships within their own group. Like Gresham, Gilkey and Zetlin question the wisdom and effectiveness of mainstreaming on these grounds.

There is also a hidden assumption that dispersal of people with disabilities within the community will raise their self-esteem by enabling them to feel better, more valued or more 'normal' about themselves. Although Wolfensberger does not mention self-esteem (Briton 1979), without some such reference to subjective self-experience normalisation sounds hollow. Equally, O'Brien's (1981, 1987) accomplishment 'respect' is supposed to include self-respect and self-esteem. However, social comparison theory (Festinger 1954) implies quite strongly that there are psychological processes which might make people with disabilities who have been dispersed feel considerably worse about themselves.

In essence, Festinger held that people have a drive to evaluate their opinions and abilities in comparison with others. Given a range of possible figures to compare him- or herself against, the individual will tend to choose someone close to his or her ability and opinions. This is because it is very difficult to compare oneself with others who are very different. The net result is that individuals choose to affiliate with others like themselves; this effect is even more pronounced when people are in situations which generate stress (Cottrell and Epley 1977). A stressful situation for someone with learning difficulties could well be interaction with non-handicapped others (Reiss and Benson 1984; Levine 1985). Put bluntly, unless strenuous and sensitive efforts are made to prevent it, people with disabilities in an integrated setting may find themselves in a situation in which a large proportion of the social comparisons they make will merely serve to confirm in them a sense of inferiority.

There is not a large body of research on social comparisons and people with learning difficulties; however, there is evidence that they can and do compare themselves with others (Coleman 1983; Gibbons 1985; Oliver 1986). Coleman's study is of particular interest since it highlights the mistakes that can be made in inferring what another person will think or feel in a given situation. He asked children with learning difficulties in various educational placements (integrated, partially integrated and segregated) to complete the Piers–Harris Self Esteem Questionnaire (Piers and Harris 1964); and also asked the children's mothers to complete the same questionnaire, answering as they thought their child would answer. The result was that the children in segregated and partially segregated classes had better self-esteem than those in completely integrated classes; this was interpreted as due to the fact that, unlike the integrated children, the segregated and partially segregated children were able to make many social comparisons with similar peers which enhanced their self-esteem. However, the self-esteem questionnaires answered by the mothers gave the opposite result: mothers whose children were in segregated settings believed that such settings would have adverse effects on their children's self-esteem, presumably because they believed that the children would feel stigmatised as a result of their special class placements, or perhaps they, as mothers, felt stigmatised by having a child in a special class.

Szivos (1989) confirmed that the experience of stigma was correlated with experiencing oneself as inferior to significant comparison figures, rather than with a particular type of placement. Students with learning difficulties did select friends whom they viewed as like themselves, and found situations of enforced comparison (such as with 'superior' younger siblings) distressing. At the very least, these findings imply that a range of comparison groups need to be available to people with disabilities to enable them to develop and maintain a sense of self-worth.

The same arguments which serve to temper one's enthusiasm for integrated school settings could be used in the work environment. Despite the potential for paid work to enhance a person's perceived (and by reflection, self-perceived) worth, people with disabilities may be ostracised (Keyes 1959), and marginalised (Dijkstra 1982; Edgerton 1967). Szivos (1989) found that the experience of work carried another kind of barb: special class adolescents with learning difficulties who had had work experience tended to have higher and more normative aspirations than their peers who had not had work experience, but they did not feel themselves any more likely to be able to attain these aspirations.

As indicated earlier, there are many good reasons why disabled and non-disabled people should mix and understand each other; but this discussion leads inescapably to the conclusion that, contrary to what Wolfensberger (1972) said about our need to 'train the handicapped not to commute and recreate in groups' (54), people with disabilities may have much to gain from each others' company, and we should not be too surprised if some of them choose to do so away from the company of non-disabled people.

COMMUNITY INTEGRATION

Unless the old patterns of segregation are to be repeated, social integration must be an essential component of community care. The 'official' view, from the normalisation perspective, is that interaction with non-disabled people is a more important goal than interaction with disabled people. Wolfensberger (1983, 1988b) is explicit about the superiority of relationships with unpaid rather than paid carers and O'Brien (1981) includes community presence and community integration as two of his five service accomplishments.

As understood here, social integration will be taken to include two major factors: relationships with others, and use of community resources. Without denying that disabled and non-disabled individuals are capable of sharing warm relationships, it is important not to over-idealise the supports that disabled people can expect from either the paid or unpaid others who interact with them. There is likely to be considerable social distance between service users and staff (Bercovici 1981); and individuals with low self-esteem may feel particularly uneasy about entering into equal relationships with professionals (Szivos 1989), preferring instead to associate with others who share their stigmatised position. This has the function of providing favourable social comparisons and maintaining a comparatively positive sense of themselves.

Carers, whether paid or unpaid, may find themselves in a double bind of support and control, described by Clarke (1982):

> As regards support, the problem is that the responsible agency is unlikely to have the range of skills necessary to develop the individual's competence in all the areas necessary for him or her to gain autonomy. Hence on the one hand there is inadequate support, with the result that the individual suffers the consequences of his or her incompetence; and on the other supervision is exercised by one agent who inevitably becomes an authority figure and is driven to remedy the consequences of the individual's continuing incompetence by restrictive and coercive measures . . .
>
> (Clarke 1982: 467)

Where the responsible agency is also expected to fulfil the role of friend, the double bind may become more invidious and irresolvable: carers feeling most comfortable with a friendship role may find themselves undermined when they experience difficulty in exercising appropriate authority; conversely, a carer who, working within a hierarchical structure, feels more comfortable as an authority figure, may find it difficult to relax this authority enough to enable the person to develop the assertiveness necessary to enter into a warm and equal relationship. Such dynamics are not restricted to paid carers: Edgerton (1967) describes many of the people in his study as acquiring benefactors, people who take a paternalistic stance towards them. The convenience of such relationships may or may not outweigh the perceived loss of autonomy and self-confidence they imply: certainly, a number of Zetlin and Turner's (1984) study members greatly resented being the unequal partner in decision-making relationships with parents.

These processes, coupled with the dispersal of people with disabilities throughout the community, can lead to social isolation and loneliness. For instance, Locker *et al.* (1981) found that over a two-year period, only 6 per cent of neighbours had visited the hostel or knew a resident, and only 2 per cent had been visited by a resident. Out of McConkey *et al.*'s (1981) sample of adults living at home, only a fifth had non-disabled friends. Donegan and Potts (1988) describe their sample as 'living on the fringes of society'. Zetlin and Turner (1984) found that many of their respondents had experienced rejection by non-disabled peers. Gollay *et al.* (1979) concluded their chapter on friendships with:

> Nearly one quarter of the mentally retarded persons had no special person outside the home to turn to in a personal crisis or simply for friendship. This may be the one 'service' which a community cannot provide, but which marks the difference between the retarded person's isolated, lonely existence in the community and a life which derives meaning from the sense of belonging and being cared *about* rather than solely being cared *for*.
>
> (Gollay *et al.* 1979: 112)

Another important psychological process affecting integration may be the awareness of being stigmatised. There is considerable evidence that people with learning difficulties experience stigma as an awareness of being different from others and of being treated differently from them (see Edgerton and Sabagh 1962; Edgerton 1967; Flynn and Knussen 1986; Jahoda *et al.* 1988; Gilkey and Zetlin 1987; Koegel and Edgerton 1982; Reiss and Benson 1984; Valpey 1982; Zetlin and Turner 1984). An invidious consequence of being stigmatised is that people may attempt to disaffiliate themselves from the group who share their devalued status, and become unable to value relationships within that group. For instance, Gibbons (1985) found that when shown photographs of people independently matched for attractiveness, who had purportedly either attended a special or an ordinary school, people with learning difficulties rated the people described as handicapped as less socially skilled than the non-handicapped, less physically attractive, and less desirable as a dating or marriage partner. Oliver (1986) found a similar tendency to denigrate handicapped peers. This 'group concept problem', as Gibbons termed it, means that people with learning difficulties tend not to be attracted to others with handicaps despite the fact that these peers may form the most likely pool of potential friends and partners. Zetlin and Turner (1984) similarly found that despite having been rejected by non-handicapped peers, many of

The limits to integration? 125

their study members were not accepting of other people with learning difficulties. The result is greatly impoverished opportunities for social contact.

There is a further tension between 'passing' and 'coming out'; that is, should individuals attempt to conceal their disability and run the risk of being discredited in an uncontrolled, possibly embarrassing, situation, or should they acknowledge their status at the beginning of a relationship or interaction, and risk an unfriendly response? Edgerton (1967) describes this dilemma as 'a constantly changing balance between highly rationalized denial and gnawing self-doubt' (1967: 171). Szivos (1989) describes a young woman who felt embarrassed at joining an evening class because she felt that somehow her learning difficulty 'showed' and that people would 'know' without her telling them. This same young woman said she had never talked about this with anyone because she was afraid that if she admitted her disability to anyone they would reject her as a friend, even if they had already formed a relationship.

These processes provide a powerful explanation of the limited use of community resources by people with learning difficulties which does not rely on a model of diminished competence or individual difficulties. Few of Cheseldine and Jeffree's (1981) and only a third of McConkey et al.'s (1981) subjects took part in community activities. Most of Intagliata et al.'s (1981) subjects used community facilities only when accompanied by carers or other supervising adults. Gollay et al. (1979) found that many of their study members bemoaned their lack of freedom, although some tangential evidence suggests that this desire for freedom may be an ambivalent one based in part on a desire to appear 'normal'. Over half of Gollay et al.'s sample felt lack of self-confidence to be a problem. In Birenbaum and Re's (1979) sample, service users wanted staff to exercise more, not less control over social outings and interactions. It may be that many people with learning difficulties are frightened by lack of structure in their lives and the lack of security this represents (Brickey et al. 1982; Burkhard and Goldman 1982; Willer and Intagliata 1982). The fears voiced by Edgerton's (1967) and Gollay et al.'s (1979) study members that they will be attacked or robbed may represent further violations of these security needs.

To conclude this section, many of the assumptions about community integration contained within normalisation may be potentially erroneous and damaging. Dispersal within the community does not guarantee that people will learn to behave in a way which will overcome intolerance towards them. Instead people may feel increasingly stigmatised and cut off by social distance from non-disabled people while being physically separated from others who share their difficulties.

BUILDING A POSITIVE SOCIAL IDENTITY

When, in 1983, Wolfensberger adopted the term social role valorisation to replace normalisation and stated that 'the creation of valued roles is the highest normalisation goal', it looked as though he intended that society should replace its negative conception of disability with a positive one which valued difference, rather than conformity to social norms. However, his writings never quite fulfil this early promise. It is most telling that nowhere is disability spoken of as something which could be valued or accepted in its own right, nor are people who have disabilities able to be valued because of these qualities. Instead, social role valorisation did not mean the creation of something new, but merely the enhancing of people's skills and images all over again, to bring them into line with valued social norms. Indeed, the conservatism corollary (1983) implies bringing people up to exceptionally high standards, as does Wolfensberger's discussion about choice, in which he advocates limiting the choices of people with disabilities to a narrow range of uncontroversial and seemingly high-status options which he describes as the '*supra*-normative range of the continuum of highly valued options' (emphasis added).

By focusing on bringing people up to highly valued social norms, Wolfensberger shows that the conception of difference/deviance underlying normalisation is that of something essentially negative and something to be eliminated. The nearest he gets to valuing difference (1988a) is when he delineates a series of attributes that people with learning difficulties are supposed to possess, 'beautiful "heart qualities" ' (63), like giving warmth, spontaneity, responsiveness and trust, and so on. While not denying that many individuals with disabilities are spontaneous, responsive and trusting, such designations smack of ascribing yet another set of supra-normative values and attributes on to them so that they fulfil the role of a sort of laicised saint. This is reminiscent of the way in which previous eras have attributed the roles of 'holy innocent' or 'eternal child' to them (Wolfensberger 1969).

Herein lies one of the central contradictions of normalisation in that while it purports to revalue people with disabilities, it is rooted in a hostility to and denial of 'differentness'. From it flow ambiguous goals such as 'independence' which may be viewed with ambivalence by some people with disabilities. Corbett (1989) questions how far a person's quality of life is enhanced by making them spend monotonous hours practising skills which may never be attained to a degree which affords him or her genuine pleasure at their mastery. Similarly, paid and meaningful work is one of the cornerstones of normalisation theory (Wolfensberger 1972), and there is no doubt that work affords many people status, self-definition, respect and power, both in their own eyes and reflected through those of others. Yet many people with disabilities are marginalised at work (Dijkstra 1982; Edgerton 1967) and are not allowed to earn more than a few pounds a week for fear of losing benefits paid to them by virtue of their being 'unfit to work'. Even if our present benefit system were to change to enable people to take advantage of the monotonous and low-paid jobs that are likely to be available to them, it is highly questionable how positive the experience of such work would be. People with disabilities who are unemployed and who work at home, as do many women, may have a similar interest in redefining the status that the terms 'employed' or 'unemployed' confer on them (see Brown and Smith, this volume).

Normalisation, because it persists in denying difference, or viewing it negatively, may entrap the individual in a constant cycle of dealing with stigma: encouraging individuals to 'pass', to disaffiliate from their peer group and suffer the loneliness involved, and to put up with discriminating job opportunities because a poorly paid job is at least more highly valued than nothing at all. Yet 'passing' is but one of the options available to stigmatised groups. An alternative, described by Tajfel (1981), involves creating a separate group identity for the group and re-evaluating its hitherto negatively perceived characteristics. The positive assertion of sisterhood for the women's movement, of gayness for homosexuals and the proud slogan 'Black is beautiful' for the black movement are all examples of groups asserting their value outside the ethnocentric and patriarchal value-systems of mainstream culture.

It may also be significant that when we refer to 'people with disabilities' we are implicitly devaluing the attribute that is salient in that particular context by relegating it to the status of an almost unmentionable after-thought. Would we now use the apologetic phrasing of 'people who are black' or 'people who are female' when we have the proud assertions 'black people', 'women' or 'sisters'? I think not. Perhaps it is too soon to envisage a similar slogan of 'slow is beautiful'; after all, it is noteworthy that all the movements referred to above have chosen their own particular term to rally around, rather than the pejorative terms used to refer to them by members of the advantaged group. This underlies the importance of listening to devalued groups and according them the respect of using the labels they choose for themselves. However, we should also ask whether in denying labels we are also denying and devaluing difference. The People First statement, 'We may be handicapped but we're still people', goes some of the way towards providing a suitable affirmation of worth, but is a compensatory rather than a positive assertion of value. The option of building a positive group identity holds the exciting prospect of re-evaluating the group from within, rather than waiting for the holders of social power to confer value as and when they think fit, and conditional upon the disadvantaged group members fulfilling mainstream norms and values (cf. Brown and Smith 1989).

NORMALISATION: WHERE DO WE GO FROM HERE?

Many good things have emerged from normalisation: the emphasis on decent standards of living, and the recognition of the importance of unconscious processes connecting imagery and behaviours towards differentness. However, amid the good, there are two related aspects which must be questioned: the assumption that assimilation ('passing') into mainstream culture works or is necessarily a good thing; and the assumption that to be attributed value, disadvantaged groups should aspire to fulfil society's idealised norms. These assumptions seem to promote an essentially negative conception of differentness, thereby making it impossible to avoid disaffiliation, derogation and shame. One of the cruellest aspects of stigmatised identity is that it makes it so difficult to value friendships with other stigmatised group members; normalisation does little or nothing to redress this. As Brown and Smith (1989) put it, it is still the advantaged group which defines what is and is not to be valued. Second, because passing is an option which is essentially pursued at an individualistic level, normalisation also makes it difficult to engage in group activity to renegotiate value and status in society. Yet as Burns and Roberts (1988) point out, it may be spurious to talk about individualizing services for people with disabilities before they have learned to pursue collective action as a group.

There are similarities with both the black and the feminist movements: in the early days of consciousness raising, black people were motivated to straighten their hair and lighten their skin, and women to burn their bras and act like 'honorary men' as a symbolic gesture to assert their equal rights with the privileged class of white men. These two movements appear to have entered a new phase, which in feminism is sometimes called postfeminism, in which the groups can feel a certain pride in affirming their separateness from the white culture and the male ethic. Normalisation seems to be at the first stage of asserting equal rights, and while there is still much to be done in this area for people who are denied equal status and opportunities, the lessons learned from the black and feminist movement are that the conviction that one's group is worth fighting for has to come at least partly from within. The alternative is to wait passively for the advantaged group to confer limited equality which does not essentially alter the status quo, and which it may be motivated to avoid (Taylor and McKirnan 1984).

Because, unlike the option of passing, consciousness raising does not take place at an individual level but rather through a group, this has some profound implications for the ways in which services might change their ways of operating with disabled people. On a theoretical level, it implies questioning the assumption that dispersal within the community is necessarily a good thing. On a practical level, it means that practitioners, instead of asking the question 'does this make my client conform to valued social norms?', might ask the new question 'does this intervention improve the self concept of my client by acknowledging his or her right to feel positively about being different'? The option that is most enhancing to a person's sense of group solidarity and self-esteem may not necessarily be the most valued option. Examples of such options could include joining a group of people with disabilities for leisure activities or sheltered work; recognising the individual's right to rebel against the efficient drive towards independence implied by normalisation; or forming a group for service users and carers actively to explore the personal meaning of disability and its positive as well as negative aspects.

In this I would by no means wish to advocate a return to segregation, nor to suggest that services should cease to strive for community integration. Nor does this critique downplay the tremendous gains made by some disability services working under the aegis of normalisation. What I do want to do is to highlight some of the psychological processes such as social comparison and affiliation which pose a challenge to community integration and to the ideology of normalisation, and to encourage practitioners to think about sensitive ways in which these issues can be taken into account.

REFERENCES

Abel, T.M., and Kinder, E. (1942) *The Subnormal Adolescent Girl*, New York: Columbia University Press.

Abraham, C. (1989) 'Supporting people with a mental handicap in the community: A social psychological perspective', *Disability, Handicap and Society* 4, 2: 121–30.

Allen, P., Pahl, J., and Quine, L. (1988) *Staff in the Mental Handicap Services: A study of change*, University of Kent, Canterbury: Health Services Research Unit.

Archer, J., and Gruenberg, E.M. (1982) 'The chronically mentally disabled and "deinstitutionalization" ', *Annual Review of Psychology* 13: 445–68.

Audit Commission (1986) *Making a Reality of Community Care: A Report*, London: HMSO.

Balla, D.A. (1976) 'Relationship of institution size to quality of care: A review of the literature', *American Journal of Mental Deficiency* 81, 2: 117–24.

Baroff, G.S. (1981) 'On size and quality of residential care: A second look', *Mental Retardation* 18, 3: 113–17.

Bercovici, S. (1981) 'Quantitative methods and cultural perspectives in the study of deinstitutionalization', in H.R. Bruininks, C.E. Meyer, B.B. Sigford, and K.C. Larkin (eds) *Deinstitutionalization and Community Placement of Mentally Retarded People*, University of Minnesota: Monograph of the American Association on Mental Deficiency.

Birenbaum, A., and Re, M.A. (1979) 'Resettling mentally retarded adults in the community – almost four years later', *American Journal of Mental Deficiency* 83, 4: 323–9.

Braddock, D. (1981) 'Deinstitutionalization of the retarded: Trends in public policy', *Hospital and Community Psychiatry* 32(a): 607–15.

Brickey, M., Browning, L., and Campbell, K. (1982) 'Vocational histories of sheltered workshop employees placed in projects with industry and competitive jobs', *Mental Retardation* 20, 2: 52–7.

Briton, J. (1979) 'Normalization: What of and what for?', *Australian Journal of Mental Retardation* 5: 224–9.

Brown, H., and Smith, H. (1989) 'Whose "ordinary life" is it anyway?', *Disability, Handicap and Society* 4, 2: 105–19.

Burkhard, J.S., and Goldman, R. (1982) 'The right to be retarded', *Milieu Therapy* 2, 1: 38–44.

Burns, J., and Roberts, T. (1988) 'A feminist perspective on the normalization principle', *Psychology of Women Newsletter*, British Psychological Society, Autumn: 12–17.

Cheseldine, S.E., and Jeffree, D.H. (1981) 'Mentally handicapped adolescents: Their use of leisure', *Journal of Mental Deficiency Research* 25: 49–59.

Clarke, M. (1982) 'Where is the community which cares?', *British Journal of Social Work* 12: 453–69.

Coleman, J.M. (1983) 'Handicapped labels and instructional segregation: Influences on children's self concepts versus the perceptions of others', *Learning Disability Quarterly* 6, 1: 3–11.

Corbett, J. (1989) 'The quality of life in the "Independence" curriculum', *Disability, Handicap and Society* 4, 2: 3–11.

Cottrell, N.B., and Epley, S.W. (1977) 'Affiliation, social comparison and socially mediated stress reduction', in J.M. Suls and R.L. Miller (eds) *Social Comparison Processes*, London: John Wiley and Sons.

Dijkstra, A. (1982) 'The cost of being visibly handicapped', *International Journal of Rehabilitation Research* 5, 4: 519–41.

Donegan, C., and Potts, M. (1988) 'People with a mental handicap living alone in the community: A pilot study of their quality of life', *British Journal of Mental Subnormality* 66, 34, 1: 10–21.

Edgerton, R.B. (1967) *The Cloak of Competence: Stigma in the lives of the mentally retarded*, San Francisco: University of California Press.

Edgerton, R.B., and Sabagh, G. (1962) 'From mortification to aggrandizement: Changing self concepts in the careers of the mentally retarded', *Psychiatry* 25: 262–73.

Education Act (1981) Department of Education and Science Circular 8/81.

Education for all Handicapped Children Act (1975) PL 94–142.

Festinger, L. (1954) 'A theory of social comparison processes', *Human Relations* 7: 117–40.

Flynn, M., and Knussen, C. (1986) 'What it means to be labelled "mentally handicapped" ', *Social Work Today* 16 June 16: 11.

Gibbons, F.X. (1985) 'Stigma perception: Social comparisons among mentally retarded persons', *American Journal of Deficiency* 90, 1: 98–106.

Gilkey, G.L.-M. and Zetlin, A.G. (1987) 'Peer relations of mentally handicapped adolescent pupils at an ordinary school', *British Journal of Mental Subnormality* 64, 33, 1: 50–6.

Goffman, E., (1982) *Asylums*, Harmondsworth: Penguin.

Gollay, E., Freedman, R., Wyngaarden, M., and Kurtz, N.R. (1979) *Coming Back: The community experiences of mentally retarded people*, Cambridge, Massachusetts: Abt Books.

Gresham, F.M. (1982) 'Misguided mainstreaming: the case for social skills training with handicapped children', *Exceptional Children* 48, 5: 422–33.

Gresham, F.M. (1985) 'The utility of cognitive-behavioral procedures for social skills training with children: A critical review', *Journal of Abnormal Psychology* 13: 411–23.

Griffiths Report (1988) *Community Care: Agenda for action* – A Report to the Secretary of State for Social Services, London: HMSO.

Intagliata, J., Crosby, N., and Neider, L. (1981) 'Foster family care for mentally retarded people: A qualitative overview', in R.H. Bruininks, C.E. Meyers, B.B. Sigford, and K.C. Larkin, (eds) *Deinstitutionalization and Community Adjustment of Mentally Retarded People,* University of Minnesota: Monograph of the American Association on Mental Deficiency.

Jahoda, A., Markova, I., and Cattermole, M. (1988) 'Stigma and the self concept of people with a mild mental handicap', *Journal of Mental Deficiency Research* 32: 103–15.

Jay Report (1979) *Report of the Committee of Inquiry into Mental Handicap Nursing and Care*, Cmnd. 7468, London: HMSO.

Keyes, D. (1959) *Flowers for Algernon*, London: Cassell.

Koegel, P., and Edgerton, R.B. (1982) 'Labeling and perception of handicap among black mildly retarded adults', *American Journal of Mental Deficiency* 90, 1: 266–76.

Landesman-Dwyer, S., Sackett, G.P., and Kleinman, J.S. (1980) 'Relationship of size to resident and staff behaviour in small community residences', *American Journal of Mental Deficiency* 5, 1: 6–17.

Levine, H.G. (1985) 'Situational anxiety and everyday life experiences of mildly mentally retarded adults', *American Journal of Mental Deficiency* 90, 1: 27–33.

Lippman, L. (1977) 'Normalization and related concepts: Words and ambiguities', *Child Welfare* 56, 5: 301–10.

Locker, D., Rao. B., and Weddell, J.M. (1981) 'The impact of community care', *Apex* 9, 3: 92–3.

McConkey, R., McCormack, B., and Naughton, M. (1983a) 'A national survey of young people's perceptions of mental handicap', *Journal of Mental Deficiency Research* 27: 171–83.

McConkey, R., McCormack, B., and Naughton, M. (1983b) 'Changing young people's perceptions of mentally handicapped adults', *Journal of Mental Deficiency Research* 27: 279–90.

McConkey, R., Walsh, T., and Mulcahy, M. (1981) 'The recreational pursuits of mentally handicapped adults', *International Journal of Rehabilitation Research* 4, 4: 493–9.

McNamara, J. (1978) 'Community: A place of space and mystery', *Community Care* September (20): 20–2.

Mansell, J., Felce, D., Jenkins, J., DeKock U., and Toogood, S. (1987) *Developing Staffed Housing for People with Mental Handicaps*, Tunbridge Wells: Costello.

Nirje, B. (1960) 'The normalization principle and its human management implications', in R.B. Kugel and W. Wolfensberger (eds) *Changing Patterns in Services for the Mentally Retarded*, Washington, D.C.: Presidential Committee on Mental Retardation.

Nirje, B. (1972) 'The right to self determination', in W. Wolfensberger *The Principle of Normalization in Human Services*, Toronto: National Institute on Mental Retardation.

O'Brien, J. (1981) *The Principle of Normalisation: A foundation for effective Services*, Adapted for CMH by A. Tyne, London: CMH/CMHERA.

O'Brien, J. (1987) 'A guide to life style planning', in B. Wilcox and G.T. Bellamy (eds) *A Comprehensive Guide to the Activities Catalogue: An alternative curriculum for youth and adults with severe disabilities*, Baltimore: Paul H. Brookes.

Oliver, C. (1986) 'Self concept assessment: A case study', *Mental Handicap* 14: 24–5.

Pahl, J., and Quine, L. (1987) 'Families with mentally handicapped children', in J. Orford (ed.) *Coping with Disorder in the Family*, London: Croom Helm.

Piers, E.V., and Harris, D. (1964) 'Age and other correlates of self concept in children', *Journal of Educational Psychology* 55: 91–5.

Reiss, S., and Benson, B. (1984) 'Awareness of negative social conditions among mentally retarded, emotionally disturbed outpatients', *American Journal of Psychiatry* 141, 1: 88–90.

Ryan, J., and Thomas, F. (1980) *The Politics of Mental Handicap*, Harmondsworth: Penguin Books.

Scheerenberger, R.C. (1974) 'A model for deinstitutionalization', *Mental Retardation* Dec.: 3–7.

Stevenson, C.L. (1944) *Ethics and Language*, New Haven, CT: Yale University Press.

Szivos, S.E. (1989) 'The Self Concept of People with a Mental Handicap', Exeter: Ph.D. Thesis, University of Exeter.

Tajfel, H. (1981) *Human Groups and Social Categories*, Cambridge: Cambridge University Press.

Taylor, D.M., and McKirnan, D.J. (1984) 'A five-stage model of intergroup relations', *British Journal of Social Psychology* 83: 291–300.

Thomas, D. (1983) 'Realising the potential', *Community Care* June (30): 14–16.

Tyne, A. (1978) *Looking at Life in a Hospital, Hostel or Home or Unit*, CMH Publications.

Valpey, D.D. (1982) 'The psychological impact of eighteen years in a board and care home', *Journal of Community Psychology* 10: 95–7.

White Paper (1989) *Caring for People*, London: HMSO.

Willer, B., and Intagliata, J. (1982) 'Comparison of family care and group homes as alternatives to institutions', *American Journal of Mental Deficiency* 86, 6: 588–95.

Wolfensberger, W. (1969) 'The origin and nature of our institutional models', in R.B. Kugel and W. Wolfensberger, *Changing Patterns in Residential Services for the Mentally Retarded*, Washington: President's Committee on Mental Retardation.

Wolfensberger, W. (1972) *The Principle of Normalization in Human Services*, Toronto: National Institute on Mental Retardation.

Wolfensberger, W. (1980) 'A brief overview of the principle of normalisation', in R.J. Flynn and K.E. Nitsch (eds) *Normalization, Social Integration and Community Services*, Baltimore: University Park Press.

Wolfensberger, W. (1983) 'Social Role Valorisation: A proposed new term for the principle of Normalization', *Mental Retardation* 21, 6: 234–9.

Wolfensberger, W. (1984) 'A reconceptualization of normalization as social role valorization', *Mental Retardation* 34, 2: 22–6.

Wolfensberger, W. (1988a) 'Common assets of mentally retarded people that are commonly not acknowledged', *Mental Retardation* 26, 2: 63–70.

Wolfensberger, W. (1988b) 'Reply to "All people have personal assets" ', *Mental Retardation* 26, 2: 75–6.

Wolfensberger, W., and Thomas, S. (1983) *PASSING: Normalization Criteria and Ratings Manual* (2nd Edition), Toronto: National Institute on Mental Retardation.

Zetlin, G., and Turner, L.T. (1984) 'Self perspectives on being handicapped: Stigma and adjustment', in R.B. Edgerton (ed.) *Lives in Process: Mildly retarded adults in a large city*, Monograph No. 6, American Association on Mental Deficiency.

9 Promoting race equality through normalisation

Peter Ferns

Normalisation has recently been established as an important set of guiding principles in shaping human services in this country. However, the principles have been implemented and interpreted in many different ways and, as other chapters demonstrate, the principles have sometimes been misused, abused and subverted to fashion a humane mask for oppressive services. This chapter will explore how normalisation can be more effective in improving the lives of Black people with disabilities in an inherently racist society. The term 'Black' is used here in the political sense in that it is applicable to all people from ethnic backgrounds where the majority of people in their ethnic group have a different skin colour from 'white' people. 'Black' refers to people who have a common experience of white racism and is intended to confirm political solidarity between people on this basis.

Since normalisation was first introduced it has been unclear how these useful and important principles could be applied in a racist society. Cultural values are key factors in the implementation of service actions which are proposed by normalisation. What effect does racism have on the cultural values of the dominant white group in their transactions with less powerful and oppressed groups? There are many definitions of racism but these can be understood in terms of three basic elements. First, a pseudo-scientific ideology based on the belief that 'white races' are inherently superior to 'Black races' resulting in powerful negative stereotypes of Black people. Second, a tradition of differential power between Black and white groups of people in society and the abuse of this power by white people to disempower Black people. Third, the institutionalisation of this oppressive power resulting in a pattern of widespread discrimination against Black people on personal and institutional levels in society. The concept of different races has no scientific or biological basis and is essentially a social construction (Banton and Harwood 1975). Racism is a dynamic and complex force in society which takes many forms, most of which are covert and inherently part of fundamental societal structures. As a result, well-meaning 'professional' service providers who are unaware of racism can easily collude with institutional racism and compound its effects on the lives of Black people with disabilities.

Normalisation offered new ways forward for disability services. These human services have traditionally been based on the power of professionals to define others as 'clients':

> the power to label people as deficient and declare them in need is the basic tool for control and oppression in modern industrialized societies of democratic and totalitarian persuasions. The agents with comprehensive labelling power in these societies are the helping professionals. Their badge bestows the caring authority to declare their fellow citizens 'clients' – a class of deficient people in need.
>
> (J. McKnight, undated)

The normalisation philosophy seeks to redress the balance by switching the focus away from individual inadequacy to the social processes which operate to devalue service users. Normalisation and its associated service assessment tools seek to provide a framework for the critical analysis of human services through a structured evaluation process which could be of enormous benefit to all devalued people. However, for it to have a real impact on human services there needs to be a broader acknowledgement and analysis of power and oppression as this affects the lives of service users. Normalisation alone does not provide adequate social, economic and political analyses for it to make sense of the lives of Black service users. Normalisation must therefore explicitly promote race equality if it is going to be a viable guide to service provision in a multi-racial society.

In order to understand how normalisation could promote race equality, clarification is needed of how oppression affects various groups of people in different ways. People continually equate all oppressions, as being similar, in a simplistic and dangerous manner. It is true that oppression can manifest itself in recurrent social processes on a basic level, such as stereotyping, but its causation and effects are crucially different for Black people, people with disabilities and people with mental health problems. It is essential to understand the differences and similarities, if these overlapping forms of oppression are to be effectively tackled in relation to these groups of people.

First, considering race and disability, it is essential to state that being Black is not a disability. Disability refers to a range of physical, intellectual or emotional impairments which mar what is considered to be 'normal' functioning. People would not ordinarily actively prefer to be 'disabled' in our culture but the vast majority of Black people do actively prefer to be Black. Moreover, those few Black people who do not prefer to be Black have been affected by the powerful influence of racist images in our society. The oppression of disabled people is not caused by the person's disability in itself but by the social constructions created in response to disability. Of course there are practical problems created for an individual, say through the absence of a limb or the absence of sight. However, it is the consequent stigmatisation, stereotyping, restriction of life opportunities and attacks on self-worth which create oppression for the person concerned. Viewing a person by focusing primarily on their disabilities locks them into a pathologising model so that they cannot escape further oppression. The same is not true of race where assessing a Black person's needs by focusing on their racial identity can be desirable and constructive.

The oppression of people with disabilities occurs across different cultures and ethnic groups, it manifests itself in different ways, but is present in all cultures. It is essential critically to examine these differing social responses if environments are to be adapted to meet the needs of people with disabilities or peoples' attitudes to disability are to be changed. It is also essential to address the issue of the powerlessness of people with disabilities in our society and the ways in which they can be empowered to challenge this.

As stated before, prejudice, stereotyping and discrimination against Black people has been based on a pseudo-scientific ideology of racism which has consistently exerted a powerful influence over Western societies during the past few hundred years. Consequently, the exploitation of Black people has become institutional, diverse and covert. A recent parallel and closely allied ideology applied to disabled people was the Eugenics movement. Francis Galton (one of the founders of the 'science' of Eugenics), for instance, believed that 'the average intellectual standard of the negro race is some two grades below our own' (Fryer 1984). However, Eugenics did not have the same world-wide effects as racism in political, economic and social terms. Furthermore, the history of exploitation and oppression of Black people is illuminated by their binding social networks of family and community together with the continuity of cultural traditions shaped by oppression, resistance and the dynamic force of political awareness.

People with disabilities have had similar experiences of exploitation, abuse and extermination. However, people with disabilities were effectively segregated from society and did not have similar social networks and cultural traditions to draw upon. In the bleak and restricted conditions of the institution there were no opportunities for a consistent culture of resistance to be built up. The absence of knowledge of oppression across generations prevented a political awareness developing out of people's own experiences. Disabled people who remained in communities were often socially segregated by family and society. Their experience was one of individualised oppression with no opportunities to develop a sense of group identity with other disabled people. It is only recently that people with disabilities have become politically aware and so begun to organise themselves to demand more power. This process has been helped by de-institutionalisation and the growth of self-advocacy and user groups.

People with mental health problems also share a different culture of oppression. While physical disability implies an impairment in the functioning of the body which leads to societal responses that create oppression for the person concerned, in the case of people with mental health problems, it is primarily their social functioning that is impaired. Mental health problems are thus social and political in nature, even if there are underlying organic or genetic factors. Medical treatment is problematical even when there is a clear organic basis to disability and the medicalisation of mental health problems presents particular difficulties as treatment becomes more associated with the 'control' side of the 'care and control' balance that is inherent in all human services. For instance, in a recent report in Birmingham of patients compulsorily detained, it was found that 8–16 per cent of the Afro-Caribbeans were diagnosed as suffering from psychosis induced by cannabis. White people or Asian people did not have this diagnosis (McGovern and Cope 1987). This clearly represents an example of the use of medical diagnosis as a tool of social control.

The medical world features strongly in the oppression of people with mental health problems as it does in the oppression of people with learning difficulties. 'Mental illness' involves judgements about people's state of mind and the appropriateness of a person's behaviour. These are essentially value judgements rooted in societal norms and can never be kept as pure scientific deliberation or medical diagnosis. Once the realm of value judgements is acknowledged in the human services, issues of power and oppression become central. The power to define someone as being 'mentally ill' and so deprive someone of their liberty is one of the most effective tools of social control in society. State power is thus harnessed and used in oppressive ways to control people who are perceived as being a threat to a traditional social order. In this way the medicalisation of mental health issues can legitimise and sanitise the use of social control by the state. Evidence suggests that this is precisely what is happening to Black people in Britain today. For instance, a study to compare the compulsory detention rates of white, Afro-Caribbean and Asian males found that in the age group 16–29, the risk of being detained under the Mental Health Act was seventeen times greater for Afro-Caribbean men compared to white men (McGovern and Cope 1987).

It is important to challenge all these types of oppression. Anti-racism cannot be about opposing racism alone and colluding with other forms of oppression. While there is always a strategic need to focus on one issue at a time, it is divisive and unnecessary to invent hierarchies of oppression. Black people with disabilities experience different types of oppression concurrently, thereby creating new and more challenging situations for human services in meeting their needs. Human services are operating in an inherently racist society where personal racism leads to stereotypical views and attitudes and institutional racism leads to widespread discrimination and oppression of Black people. Normalisation is used to describe the experience of service users in a largely apolitical way although there are undoubtedly political consequences to its analysis. As a set of principles it must take into account that white societies are racist in many covert ways and not least in their value systems and 'norms'. If there is no acknowledgement of racism or analysis that includes power dynamics between oppressor and oppressed, normalisation will be in danger of being used to maintain and collude with racism in society.

Wolfensberger defines deviancy as difference which is negatively valued. He goes on to identify three types of differences that are consistently devalued in a variety of cultures. These are:

- physical differences and bodily impairments;
- overt and covert behaviours;
- attributive identities of people such as descent, nationality, the ethnic group from which a person derives, the language he/she speaks, or even a person's caste regardless of behaviour, language etc.

(Wolfensberger 1972)

He goes on to define stigmata as 'visible or obvious signs that mark a person as being devalued or as having some *socially devalued characteristic* or identity' (my emphasis). Examples given include this list: 'physical deformities, facial scars or other disfigurements, *skin colour*, a shuffling walk, clothes that are filthy . . .' (my emphasis). This definition of deviancy and stigma continues to confuse issues of race and disability. The placing of skin colour and ethnicity in the same category as 'facial scars and other disfigurements' may be an attempt at stating a social reality in an apolitical way but, in a racist society, this kind of statement will be used to further oppress Black people.

The stigmata mentioned by Wolfensberger would not be positively valued by an overwhelming majority of people in our society regardless of their racial background. However, nearly all Black people, who represent a significant proportion of our population, positively value their skin colour and ethnicity. Moreover, on a world-wide basis, being Black and from an ethnic group where most people are Black is the 'norm'. How can this characteristic be equated with being 'facially disfigured' or 'physically deformed'?

The only reason why being a Black person is devalued in our society is because of racism. Racism is too complex to be justified on the basis of 'negatively valued difference'. Social, political and economic factors are much more influential in oppressing Black people than the largely inter-personal processes which have been the focus of deviancy theorists. Confusing negatively valued differences with ethnicity strengthens the idea that racism is inherent to all human societies, but whereas physical disability is negatively valued everywhere being Black is not. Racism in its fully developed form, based on a pseudo-scientific ideology, institutionalised differential power between 'races' and widespread discrimination on the basis of race, is most prevalent in Western societies. Its influence is so powerful and pervasive that secondary effects of white racism are even evident in countries where the majority of people are Black. Secondary effects of racism result mainly from colonialism and the earlier legacy of slavery. Examples include the skewed economies of countries that are still recovering from colonial economic exploitation and the underlying assumptions in some ex-colonial countries that Western cultures are superior to all others. Racism is primarily a white Western problem.

Wolfensberger's initial confusion in equating race and disability in his definition of deviancy and stigma is compounded when he goes on to outline two basic strategies to enable devalued persons to 'attain (more) valued membership in society'.

First, he suggests reducing the differentness or stigmata of the person concerned and, second, changing societal perceptions so that the devalued characteristics of a person are no longer viewed negatively. What are the consequences of these strategies for Black people with disabilities or other forms of 'deviancies'? The former strategy of reducing differentness or stigmata may make sense in relation to the person's disability or physical disfigurement but it is unthinkable to advocate that the colour of a person's skin or their ethnicity should be made more 'acceptable' to white society. There are, for example, skin whiteners which Black people buy in Africa and the USA in the belief that appearing more white-skinned is socially and aesthetically more desirable. It is also racist to suggest that a Black person should change their traditional dress just to reduce their 'differentness'. This strategy is clearly unacceptable where it is based on a definition of stigmata that includes skin colour or ethnicity.

Changing societal perceptions of differentness is, however, consistent with anti-racist strategies of challenging racist ideologies and stereotypes and promoting race equality. In relation to Black people with disabilities, this strategy should lead human service workers actively to challenge stereotypical views of Black people with disabilities.

Each of the Seven Core Themes of normalisation must be critically analysed and viewed from a Black perspective if a new interpretation is to be formulated which can then be usefully applied to Black people with disabilities. There follows a brief outline of how such an interpretation can be approached with some suggestions about consequences for practice.

THE ROLE OF (UN)CONSCIOUSNESS IN HUMAN SERVICES

> Normalization incorporates the explicit assumption that consciousness is preferable to unconsciousness, and that negative feelings and dynamics should, and usually have to, be made conscious in order to be adaptively addressed. Thus, normalization is extensively concerned with the identification of unconscious (usually negative) dynamics within human services that contribute to the devaluation and oppression of certain groups of people in society, and provides conscious strategies for remediating the devalued social status of such people.
>
> (Wolfensberger and Thomas 1983: 25)

This Theme would also be strongly advocated in an anti-racist approach. Anti-racism would require making the value-base of human service more explicit to enable values to be challenged and changed. Racism induces all sorts of moral panics in white, democratic societies, where the reality of its presence is difficult and unpleasant to face up to. Nowadays, the denial of racism as an unpleasant reality results in covert racism at both institutional and personal levels. The mechanisms of denial are varied, complex and dynamic in nature; they are maintained through apathy or cultural arrogance. For instance white people often do not see racism as a problem if there are few Black people living nearby or social workers may assume that 'white' child-rearing practices are best and embark on a mission to educate the 'uncivilised foreigners' on how to raise their children. Thus racist ideology permeates the structure of human services in this country. The lack of culturally sensitive services, the low take-up of services by Black people and the punitive approach taken to Black users are all manifestations of powerful, covert processes (Cheetham 1982; Gordon 1986). Services assume a 'white' norm thereby establishing white cultures as being more influential and superior to Black cultures. This has devastating effects for Black service users in that it denies their self-identity, erodes their self-confidence and causes psychological confusion about racial identity (Black and in Care Steering Group 1984; Maxime 1987). Furthermore, once white norms have been established, Black people are inevitably perceived as threats to the white status quo and are therefore more likely to be subjected to social control through state agencies including human services. An anti-racist approach would differ from normalisation in providing 'conscious strategies for remediating devalued social status'. Anti-racism would attempt to go further in tackling political and economic discrimination through policy frameworks and explicit strategies for change.

The consequences for practice implied by this Theme, include the following issues. In challenging racist ideology, careful analysis of the values underlying services must be undertaken to ensure that they are not based on racist assumptions and stereotypes of Black people. An example of this has been the resistance, until recently, of fostering and adoption agencies to recruiting Black foster parents (Small 1986) based on the racist assumption that Black families practised inferior methods of child-rearing compared to white families and a stereotypical view that Black families were not interested in fostering children. Values and norms of the service should be inclusive of all groups of people using the service. Exposing the values of a service requires explicit statement of the service's aims.

Racist practices must be acknowledged and a commitment made to the development of services that promote equality for all oppressed groups of service users. Empowerment of Black people by services would require the promotion of a sense of pride in Black peoples' history and, on an individual level, a willingness to talk to Black service users about their experiences of racism and oppression.

THE RELEVANCE OF ROLE EXPECTANCY AND ROLE CIRCULARITY TO DEVIANCY-MAKING AND DEVIANCY-UNMAKING

> When the dynamic of role expectancy is at work, a person or group of people who hold certain (possibly unconscious) expectancies about the behaviour or growth potential of another person or group will create conditions and circumstances that generally tend to elicit the expected behaviour.
>
> (Wolfensberger and Thomas 1983: 25)

The 'self-fulfilling prophecy' has affected Black people with disabilities in the way that the intellectual capabilities of Black people have been stereotyped. Cultural bias in intelligence testing and institutional racism in the educational system have resulted in many Black children being wrongly classified as having learning difficulties (Tomlinson 1981; Jenkins *et al.* 1979; Shelley and Cohen 1986).

These kinds of racist stereotypes decrease the learning opportunities for Black people with learning difficulties or physical disabilities. The exclusive promotion of white cultures inevitably leads to the strengthening of a racist devaluation of Black cultures. So, for example, the activities offered to Black service users are often culturally inappropriate and deny and invalidate their cultural expertise and skills, resulting in further devaluation of Black service users. However, people are rarely as passive as the Theme implies: Black people down through history have developed a culture of resistance and survival in the face of such expectations.

Black service users therefore may actively resist; indeed, there is some evidence to suggest that resistance by Black service users evokes a great deal more fear and hostility from white-dominated institutions than that of other service users. Black service users quickly become labelled as being aggressive or as presenting 'problem behaviours', resulting in punitive treatment by the authorities (see Burke 1986).

Practice issues arising from this Theme would involve attempts to break the process of role expectancy and role circularity. For Black service users, this would mean that services should be planned on positive expectations of Black people. Culturally appropriate activities would be offered taking into account issues of gender, religion and spirituality. (Many Eastern cultures take a more holistic approach to human needs and individual experience in terms of mind, body and spirit.) Black service users should be offered training opportunities which help them to break out of the personal limitations imposed through racist stereotypes. Services should seek to emphasise the positive contribution of Black people to society and in their local communities. There should be an expectation that service users would share in decision-making processes and planning of new services. This would entail dismantling bureaucratic systems that exclude 'non-professional' people and keep information about service provision from service users.

THE CONSERVATISM COROLLARY TO THE PRINCIPLE OF NORMALISATION

... the conservatism corollary of normalisation posits that the greater the number, severity, and/or variety of deviances or stigmata ... of an individual person, or the greater the number of deviant stigmatised persons there are in a group or setting, the more impactful it is to (a) reduce one or a few of the individual stigmata within the group, (b) reduce the proportion or number of deviant people in the group, or (c) balance (compensate for) the stigmata or deviances by the presence, or additions, of positively valued manifestations.

(Wolfensberger and Thomas 1983: 26)

Given Wolfensberger's definition of deviancy and stigma, it is an un-acceptable strategy, for Black people with disabilities, to reduce individual stigma within the group or to reduce the number of 'deviant' people in the group in terms of colour or ethnicity, while it is, of course, desirable to increase the positive value ascribed to Black people with disabilities. The Theme can therefore be abused if it is used to impose the cultural values of the majority white population on to the minority Black population. If the Theme were based on values of race equality, there would be no need to reduce differentness in cultural terms as the cultural variety of people would be valued and the Theme could not be used by people to collude with racism.

Cultural variety is beginning to be valued in society, particularly in youth cultures, and this healthy process of cultural pluralism should be actively encouraged. Advocating the reduction of differences in cultural terms runs directly counter to values of race equality which would seek to strengthen cultural diversity.

In practice, the Theme should result in the positive valuing of diversity and of the different cultures of service users. The 'highly valued means' referred to in this Theme should therefore be those which are highly valued in terms of the service user's culture since enhancement of the positive status of Black service users has to be set in the context of the Black service user's own community networks. For example, if an Asian woman with disabilities wished to get married it may well be most appropriate for an 'arranged marriage' to be pursued even though such a custom may be devalued in the majority white population. The 'conservatism corollary' would however run counter to this interpretation and employ the dominant white values inappropriately to the lives of Black users.

THE DEVELOPMENTAL MODEL AND THE IMPORTANCE OF PERSONAL COMPETENCY ENHANCEMENT

Normalisation requires that the personal competencies of people (especially if they are devalued or at risk) should be enhanced . . . the developmental model can lead to tremendous client growth because of its positive assumptions about the abilities of every person to grow, its high demands and expectancies, and its requirements that effective pedagogic techniques and adaptive equipment be used in order to help people to develop or function.

(Wolfensberger and Thomas 1983: 26)

As I have stated before, personal and institutional experiences of racism have resulted in an even greater denial of opportunities and experiences to

Black people with disabilities which hinders their growth and development. The issues raised by this Theme fit well with strategies of positive action which redress inequalities in the opportunities open to Black people to develop and to compete on an equal basis. One such strategy would be to provide special training opportunities for Black people with disabilities to learn new skills for survival and development in a racist environment. The Theme should encourage service workers to have positive attitudes towards the abilities of Black users and have high expectations of them. Black users from different cultures must be taught skills that are appropriate to their culture but services should also provide information and knowledge to Black and white service users about how racism operates in society and help Black users to develop the skills to cope with and challenge racism. White users also require skills in recognising and challenging racism. The skills and strengths of Black people with disabilities in surviving racism should be recognised and used positively. In common with all service users, Black service users may need help in developing self-advocacy skills.

THE POWER OF IMITATION

> Normalisation requires that the dynamic of imitation be capitalized upon in a positive way, especially for the benefit of devalued persons, so that the models provided to devalued persons are people who function routinely in a more appropriate, and hopefully even valued, fashion. Furthermore, normalisation implies that one would increase the sense of identification of service clients with valued models, because people are much more apt to imitate those with whom they identify.
>
> (Wolfensberger and Thomas 1983: 27)

Black people with disabilities who have entered into institutions have been even more isolated and segregated than white people because they are Black people in largely white institutions. Due to institutional racism, there is a greater lack of valued models of Black people in socially valued roles in all parts of society. This fact is reflected in human services where Black workers are often found in lower status jobs with little power or authority in the service system. Black workers are not encouraged to use their own experience and knowledge of oppression, such human resources are de-valued by 'white' professionalism.

This Theme should lead services to counteract devaluing, racist stereo-types of Black people by employing highly skilled Black staff (or by providing training opportunities for existing Black staff) to provide positive role models for Black service users. Service organisations would therefore need to have well developed equal opportunities policies in recruitment and selection of staff as well as in ensuring equality of career progression for all its workers. Services should also consciously highlight the experiences of Black people with disabilities who have successfully overcome their problems in terms of housing, employment and attaining socially valued roles in society. Black service users would thus be enabled to build social relationships with valued Black people. This would require services to work more collaboratively with Black communities than they have done in the past and as a first step to ensure that information about services is really accessible to Black communities.

THE DYNAMICS AND RELEVANCE OF SOCIAL IMAGERY

> Normalisation implies that the social image of (devalued) people be enhanced. This means that as much as is honest and possible, any features of a human service which can convey any image messages about the (devalued) clients should be positive ones . . .
>
> (Wolfensberger and Thomas 1983: 27)

A long tradition of racist stereotyping has resulted in many negative images of Black people. Current media images continue this stereotyping in more subtle forms. The media continues to portray Black people as threats to society and feed the propensity for human services to be used as a form of social control.

The practical implications of this Theme involve a recognition that Black people with disabilities are made vulnerable by racist stereotyping. The image of Black service users presented by human services should therefore be carefully scrutinised and information about services take pains to present positive images of Black people with disabilities. The physical settings provided for Black people should promote a positive image of Black cultures through the use of photographs, posters, art objects, books and so on. The physical care of Black service users should be undertaken by appropriately skilled staff and personal care materials, for example, African hair care, creams for Black skin care used to enhance service users appearance and comfort. Culturally appropriate food should be provided as a matter of course for reasons both of taste and religious requirements.

THE IMPORTANCE OF PERSONAL SOCIAL INTEGRATION AND VALUED SOCIAL PARTICIPATION

> Normalisation requires that, to the highest degree and in as many life areas as feasible, a (devalued) person or group have the opportunity to be personally integrated into the valued life of society.
>
> (Wolfensberger and Thomas 1983: 27)

In human services, Black service users often experience a greater degree of segregation than other service users. In a study at Springfield Hospital in South London it was found that in the case of 'uncooperative patients', 87 per cent of Afro-Caribbean and African patients as opposed to 36 per cent of white British patients were transferred to a 'locked ward' (Bolton 1984). Reversing this process means taking on board the issue of integrating Black people with disabilities into communities in multiracial areas as well as services. Support for Black service users living in the community must therefore include help in dealing with the increasingly common experience of racial harassment. Policy statements, clear procedures and skills training are key elements of such support.

Concern about congregation of devalued people, which is at the root of this Theme, should never be used as a rationale to stop Black people with disabilities from meeting as a group. As in the case of other Black people, Black people with disabilities need to meet as a group to strengthen their own identity, increase their self-advocacy skills and to aid their empowerment.

Normalisation has been and continues to be a powerful influence in shaping and improving human services. This chapter has not argued for its dismantling or simply dismissed the principles as being racist in nature. Normalisation does have a great deal to offer Black people with disabilities but only if it fully embraces race equality as one of its own core values. Normalisation describes key elements of a process of empowerment through enhancing positively valued social roles for people, increasing personal competencies and challenging devaluing images and stereotypes of service users which are often covert in human services. These elements of empowerment can form a basis for social and political action for Black people with disabilities if they incorporate an explicitly anti-racist approach. Normalisation challenges human services to take a critical look at their own practices and to clarify more exactly what they are achieving for people who are using services. It can be used to challenge professional power and support attempts to redress the power imbalance between those who hold power in human services and those who do not. An anti-racist perspective can sharpen up this analysis of power dynamics between the people who maintain oppression and those who are oppressed. Such an analysis can lead to a model of empowerment for individuals, their families and communities which would radically change human services that are liberal in their intentions but oppressive in their effects. As oppressive forces increase in society and become more covert, human services will only serve to collude with and maintain oppression unless we challenge these ideologies and take positive action to empower people who are vulnerable to devaluation and people whose dignity and worth is constantly being devalued. Human services have tremendous opportunities to change the lives of oppressed people and help them to realise their potential. In order to do this, normalisation must formulate anti-racist strategies for the eradication of discrimination on personal and institutional levels, for the promotion of equality for all oppressed groups in society and for the empowerment of service users. Normalisation on its own will never be applied effectively in multiracial societies unless it undergoes this trans-formation. Racism in our society has to be actively challenged and equality actively promoted because, in Malcolm X's words, 'if you're not part of the solution, you're part of the problem'. Let us hope that people working in human services can meet the challenges successfully because oppressed and devalued people cannot afford our failure.

REFERENCES

Banton, M., and Harwood, J. (1975) *The Race Concept*, London: David and Charles.

Black and in Care Steering Group (1984) 'Black and in care: Conference Report', London: Blackhorse Press.

Bolton, P. (1984) 'Management of compulsorily admitted patients to a high security unit', *International Journal of Social Psychiatry* 30: 77–84, quoted in S. Fernando, *Race and Culture in Psychiatry*, London: Tavistock/Routledge (1988).

Burke, A. (1986) 'Racism, prejudice and mental illness', in J. Cox (ed.) *Trans-cultural Psychiatry*, London: Croom Helm, 139–57.

Cheetham, J. (1982) *Social Work Services for Ethnic Minorities in Britain and USA*, London: DHSS.

Fryer, P. (1984) *Staying Power – the history of black people in Britain*, London: Pluto Press.

Gordon, P. (1986) 'Racism and Social Security', *Critical Social Policy*, 17, Autumn.

Jenkins, D., Kemmis, S., MacDonald, B., and Verma, G.K. (1979) 'Racism and educational evaluation', in G.K. Verma and C. Bagley (eds) *Race Education and Identity*, London: MacMillan, 107–32.

McGovern, D., and Cope, R. (1987) 'The compulsory detention of males of dif-ferent ethnic groups, with special reference to offender patients', *British Journal of Psychiatry* 150: 505–12.

McKnight, J. (unpublished) 'The professional problem'.

Maxime, J. (1987) 'Some psychological models of black self-concept', in S. Ahmed, J. Cheetham, and J. Small (eds) *Social Work with Black Children and their Families*, London: Batsford.

Shelley, D., and Cohen, D., (1986) *Testing Psychological Tests*, London: Croom Helm.

Small, J. (1986) 'Transracial placements: Conflicts and contradictions', in S. Ahmed, J. Cheetham, and J. Small (eds) *Social Work with Black Children and their Families*, London: Batsford.

Tomlinson, S. (1981) *Educational Subnormality – a study in decision-making*, London: Routledge and Kegan Paul.
Wolfensberger, W. (1972) *Normalization*, Toronto: NIMR.
Wolfensberger, W., and Thomas, S. (1983) *PASSING Manual* (2nd Edition), Toronto: NIMR.

10 Assertion, not assimilation
A feminist perspective on the normalisation principle

Hilary Brown and Helen Smith

We affirm the existence of all those who have for centuries been negatively defined: not only women, but the 'untouchable', the 'unmanly',
'the non-white', the 'illiterate', the invisible. Which forces us to confront the problem of the essential dichotomy: power and powerlessness.
(Rich 1986: 64)

This chapter offers a feminist perspective on normalisation, looking first at
the contribution which feminist theory can make to our understanding of
the lives of people with disabilities and second at the implications of
normalisation for women who use services, care for disabled relatives or
work in new community services. Feminist theory provides a clear analysis
of power and powerlessness that can offer depth to our understanding of the
position of people with disabilities. The difficulties of implementing high
quality services for them are not just practical, as is often suggested, but
may be rooted in the theory's failure to address alternative routes to
empowerment for groups of people who, for different reasons and with
different consequences, find themselves living on the margins.

Sceptics might argue that the position of women, especially middle-
class, articulate women, bears no resemblance to that of people with learning difficulties or mental health problems and that the application of
feminist thinking to their situation detracts from the very particular discrimination and deprivation to which they are subject. Our reasons for
drawing parallels are fourfold. First, community care policies dis-
proportionately affect women not only as users (especially of services for
elderly people) but overwhelmingly as carers and as direct care workers in
services for all client groups. Second, the recent women's movement has
been roughly contemporaneous with the normalisation movement and has
been attempting to achieve similar acceptance and improvement in the
status of its constituents. Third, the widespread moves towards deinstitutionalisation have mostly dispersed services from public organisations into

the 'private' world of caring. In its analysis of the 'personal as political', feminist theory is able to straddle the boundary between private and public forms of care and analyse the implications of public policies for the private sphere. Finally, the women's movement shares an essentially humanist commitment to the eradication of the abuse and neglect of vulnerable groups of people. Dworkin (1986) asserts that feminism is

> like other political movements in one important way. Every political movement is committed to the belief that there are certain kinds of pain that people should not have to endure. They are unnecessary. They are gratuitous. They are not part of the God given order. They are not biologically inevitable. They are acts of human will. They are acts done by some human beings to other human beings.

> (Dworkin 1986: 134).

In this respect normalisation and the feminist campaigns, against discrimination, oppression, violence and poverty, share a common core.

LINKS BETWEEN FEMINISM AND NORMALISATION

We have argued elsewhere (Brown and Smith 1989) that the manifestations of abuse and degradation which normalisation so clearly exposes in institutions for people with disabilities are not specific to them, but common expressions of power and control. Thus, for example, the pervasive use of childlike language when referring to people with learning difficulties has parallels in the pejorative use of 'boy' to address Black men or the description of adult women as 'girls'. What is being expressed and acknowledged is the power relationship between the two parties in such exchanges, what is being effected is the subordination of the person who is a member of the devalued group. In other words the notion of *de*valuation implies the existence of an individual or group who are actively exercising power over others, it is not a passive condition. These more valued individuals do the devaluing, but within normalisation they are also portrayed as models of appropriate behaviour and as the arbiters of what is valuable.

Wolfensberger's analysis of the unconscious imagery which surrounds and degrades people with disabilities (see Emerson, this volume) has parallels in the work of Dworkin (1981) who confronts the objectification of women and the juxtaposition of sex, torture and brutality in pornography. Both argue from the position that such images betray intent, that they are not, even if subliminal, harmless, but systematic in their effects on people with disabilities and on individual women. Calling a person a vegetable justifies treating the person as if they had no feelings, just as calling a woman a bitch contains within it the rights of ownership and the rationale for control. These images create a climate in which it is possible to justify individual acts of degradation or brutality, but they are also, in themselves, acts of brutality and degradation. These words and images pervade public as well as private consciousness and hence underpin public institutions and provision. They distort humanity.

Both movements initially began to fight back by believing that gaining access to the mainstream would remedy the situation, as if being marginalised had been little more than an unfortunate oversight. Wolfensberger, says Booth (1988), thought that if people simply attended to the normalisation principle, discrimination would stop; however, 'He shows no awareness of the powerful interests which are used to keep the contradictions of professional practice hidden' (Booth 1988: 104).

The normalisation movement, using its analysis of the oppressive and segregating features of institutionalisation, drew up an agenda in which these features were very precisely reversed. Thus services were charged with providing ordinary housing within ordinary neighbourhoods, with arranging activities which were in tune with those of other valued adults and conformed to the expectations which others might have of their relatives or neighbours. In doing this, many services have achieved a quantum leap in the quality of life of people with disabilities. People who had lived in barren, unwelcoming environments were now properly housed, clothed and fed. In Britain, the public scandals which erupted in the 1970s about the state of hospital accommodation and the corruption and ill-treatment endemic in them further fuelled the move to relocate services.

Thus normalisation contributed a framework designed to reverse the negative effects of institutional malpractice. The key features of this framework were the dispersal of services to avoid congregation, the siting of services 'in the community' to avoid segregation and 'image enhancement', that is, attending to the way people with disabilities present themselves to valued members of the public. The overall aim was to create valued social roles for people with disabilities, so that they could be seen as valued members of the community.

Early feminist writing similarly began by identifying that men were valued principally in their economic roles and that these held the key to public prominence and rights of decision making. Liberal feminists such as Friedan (1963) urged middle-class women to go out to work but ignored the supports that would be needed for them to do so. Childcare and housework were seen as individual problems to which individual solutions could be found if one were determined enough. The anomalous fact that these solutions involved the exploitation of working-class women and Black women was rarely discussed.

The experience of women entering the employment market has not been one of unrivalled opportunity, nor has it succeeded in earning for women, the respect of men. If anything, the trends have been in the opposite direction. Individual women seeking to enter high-status areas such as stock broking or law met with hostility, their qualifications to do the job were not welcomed or accepted, in short they were not 'allowed' to enter the field. As legislation and custom gave way and women demolished the arguments against them, for example by proving that they are competent and can lift heavy weights, the prejudice against individuals remained. Moreover, where women took valued jobs in any number, it was the status of the job which went down rather than the status of the women which went up. This continued marginalisation testifies to the direct benefits which accrue to men, both individually and as a group, from the second-class status of women in the labour market and to their ingenuity in maintaining it either overtly through discrimination, passively by not providing personal or communal support for childcare, or more covertly through an ideology in which women are portrayed as things. Wherever there are hierarchies, women are congregated at the bottom of them.

The situation for people with disabilities is different in degree but perhaps not in effect. Experience in North America suggests that people with disabilities are only gaining access in significant numbers to jobs in low-status areas with minimum wages, as demographic changes make these positions difficult to fill by non-disabled people. There are constant questions to be asked about whether such work is valued, valuable, exploitative or beneficial. People with disabilities want – and have a right to – employment but human services are often too sanguine about the nature of those jobs. For example, many boring and repetitive jobs performed by women are compensated for in part by comradeship and a sense of community, while others isolate and even endanger people. Women have learned that the costs and benefits of employment are complex and often difficult to weigh up. Alternative structures, such as co-operatives and small businesses, can provide more choice and autonomy but they do so often at the expense of financial viability. Women who, like people with disabilities; exist on the tightrope stretched between the world of work and the world of benefits, have learned to question the role of paid work as a route to valued status in the community. The disability movement may be at a similar point of revelation.

Access to employment has represented one area of campaigning for both women and people with disabilities; the other common issue of campaign has revolved around rights in the private sphere, that is, rights to homes which are safe and comfortable and in which people are cared for and able to express themselves. As Dalley argues (1988) the model which has been adopted by human services as the most valued is overwhelmingly that of small pseudo-family group homes. The large hospital reprovision such as Darenth Park (a large mental handicap hospital in south-east England) succeeded in dispersing people in small groups into the communities from which they originated; only then was attention paid to the social needs of those individuals to have contact with the people with whom they had originally lived (see *Network*, the newsletter of former residents of Darenth Park Hospital).

The evidence suggests that while such homes offer an improved quality of life they also leave people vulnerable (see Flynn 1987) and with tenuous social networks (see Atkinson and Ward 1987). It seems that, with the exception of trips to the shops, many people with disabilities are more or less confined to the home as women are when they are responsible for young children or dependent relatives. Segregation, therefore, can take place in two ways: one we have seen in the congregation of large numbers of devalued people in large communal buildings, behind fences and off the bus route; and one we may be about to witness, as the same people are isolated in ones and twos in private spaces to which others do not have access. Such isolation is made complete if people are afraid and/or unable to go out, have little money, have no places to meet others who are in the same situation and are not believed if they complain about the way they are being treated. The common feature of both forms of segregation is that individuals are under the power and/or protection of more powerful individuals whose rights to control, neglect, reward, punish, enable or restrict are unchecked.

The cumulative effect of these conditions is to render people with disabilities and their concerns, rights, achievements or suffering invisible to the wider society. A scandal in one home will not be taken as an indictment of all, it will scarcely be noticed. Feminism offers an understanding of what it feels like to be a hostage in one's own community, of how it is possible to be present but not allowed to participate, of the continuous juggling act between 'passing' (Goffman 1961) in roles which are designed by and for men, accommodating to low-status roles which are sanctioned for women and acting autonomously on the basis of one's own desires and experience.

It is this removal of the fight for improved services from the public arena to the home front which has caused us as feminists to question the imperative in normalisation to individualise service provision and reject collective solutions. If services are individualised, problems are personalised. If vulnerable people are dispersed from one another neither they, nor people working on their behalf, are able to see common threads or patterns. Opportunities for victim blaming abound: 'She was asking for it'; 'It is part of her condition'. In instances where women have collectively sought to bring issues into the public arena, for example the extent of sexual abuse against women and children, they have begun to counter the myth that such abuse is an aberration, an isolated incident to which they in some way had contributed. As a movement, women have been able to challenge the ideology (which incidentally is so pervasive that one could almost say it were culturally valued) which keeps women dependent on individual men and which sexualises violence undermining the credibility of individual women who resist or fight back (see Dworkin 1986: 273). As Dworkin asserts, whether in the context of racism, sexual orientation, gender, mental illness, learning disability or physical impairment, 'Wherever power is accessible or bodily integrity honored on the basis of biological attribute, systematized cruelty permeates the society' (Dworkin 1986: 115).

In terms of political action, congregation on one's own terms (either in places or through networks) can counter the effects of systematised inequality and return the issue to the public arena. It strengthens the visibility and the credibility of individual women who have been victimised. Movements such as Women's Aid have been a political as well as a personal success for the many women who have had need of them. They are, says Pascall (1987),

> something new. They offer essential accommodation. But they also offer help without condition or bureaucratic barrier; acceptance of women's own assessment of their need for refuge; mutual aid and community. They stand in place of bureaucratic and professional gatekeepers, hierarchy and authority – more typical characteristics of 'social services'.
>
> (Pascall 1987: 162)

The refuges also directly challenge the assumption that small, isolated family groups are the most beneficial for all who live in them. Women and children have much to gain from communal support and protection. The typical size of household groups has more to do with economics than with efficacy, the layout of neighbourhoods more to do with male town planners than women and children who primarily inhabit them. People with disabilities, with their exaggerated problems of mobility and their additional needs for support, may also be ill served by limited options for communal living.

Dworkin (1986: 266) maintains that victimisation has four elements: first there is a hierarchy; then there is objectification; then there is submission because the 'situation of that person requires obedience and compliance', or as Walmsley (1989: 5) observes of people with learning difficulties, 'they need to behave in an accommodating way ... to "obey" rather than challenge their care givers'; fourth there is violence. 'The violence', says Dworkin 'is systematic, endemic enough to be unremarkable and normative'. The normalisation movement developed in response to its recognition of the systematised abuse of institutionalised regimes but twenty years on people with disabilities are still at risk of becoming victims on all four counts. The agenda for new services must, therefore, recognise the possibility of abuse, actively reverse the expectation of submission, fight, as normalisation theory has always encouraged, the objectification of people with disabilities and resist hierarchical forms of organisation which always render service users at the bottom of the pile.

Furthermore, as women began to appreciate the ways in which culturally valued norms not only isolate them but enforce their silence, they have increasingly sought to protect some space for themselves where they can interact without having to be bound by men's dominant expectations. They do so, not only as a route to political action but as an opportunity for personal validation and empowerment. This self-segregation allows women to share their experiences, to make space for their own expression whether artistic, sporting or political, space to be safe and to set their own standards. 'Women only' cafés, libraries, publishing houses, sections of political parties, all allow women to develop the confidence to be in the world without the constraints of culturally sanctioned roles. At a personal level, such space allows women to speak and be heard.

Self-segregation thus offers primarily a place to be oneself and secondarily a forum to resist oppression. We disagree with Wolfensberger and Tullman (1989) who see any attempt at self-segregation as enforced and necessarily marginalising:

> Only a few people or groups can be said to truly and deliberately choose social marginalisation and devaluation of their own free will. Even when they say they do, they often do so only reactively in response to prior rejection by society.
>
> (Wolfensberger and Tullman 1989: 218)

We would argue that white men have always been able to self-segregate, they manage to do so even when they are with other groups of people, even when they are outnumbered! Deliberate self-segregation may be seen, not only as an explicit reactive strategy to oppression but as part of a dynamic in which devalued groups are not 'allowed' to set boundaries. Women, for example, who go out together are often accosted on the grounds that they are 'alone'. Service users are also constantly interrupted or interpreted, partly by virtue of needing help; they may also not have the requisite communication skills to forge links with each other. We would therefore add to O'Brien's (1987) list of service accomplishments (see Emerson, this volume) a requirement to seek opportunities for people with disabilities to have 'meaningful association' with others who share their oppression and for services to develop skills in protecting such association and facilitating it when, and only when, it is appropriate for them to be involved.

This is not to justify a return to block arrangements and demeaning bulk deals for people with disabilities but to highlight their need for opportunities to make links and share experiences and activities with others who have faced similar issues. Otherwise they may never see someone who has survived the system, or be able to talk at first hand about the issues or choices which may face him or her in adult life. It is to argue that people with disabilities be enabled to acknowledge their handicaps and supported as they express their pain at being different (Sinason 1986) and their distress about options which may not be open to them (see Brown 1983; Szivos and Griffiths 1990). Activities should enable individuals to share, rather than avoid, their experiences of differentness. Oliver (1988) argues that

> disabled adults must participate much more actively in the education of disabled children for it is only those people with direct experience of the special education system who can know just how disabling it can be.
>
> (Oliver 1988: 28)

The 1980s has been characterised by the emergence of distinct interest groups, self help movements and, following Tajfel's (1981) framework (see Szivos, this volume), groups which are assertively defining themselves as minority groups on account of their ethnicity, sexual orientation or particular social problems or circumstances. The gay community, facing the tragedy of Aids, throws

> into stark relief what many in the gay constituency knew already ... that a kinship based on shared nature and a consequent shared oppression can be as mutually sustaining as that of family, and in many ways more binding and less conditional.
>
> (Edgar 1987)

Weeks (1989: 130) refers to 'communities of choice' or 'elective communities'. To belong to any such group involves owning and acknowledging what it is that one has in common with the other members, to respect and value oneself alongside others who are like oneself. We have written earlier (Brown and Smith 1989) about the possible fragility of these relationships and networks, especially if the group who have come together have not been able to wrest any elements of a positive self-image from the treatment which they have received from society at large:

> Relationships between people who come together on the basis of alienation or a shared history of oppression are complex and ambivalent. People whose identity is fragile are vulnerable to competition and envy and may find it difficult to identify with each other. They see in the stigma of the other, their own degradation. They may apply the same

oppressive categories as professionals to lift themselves out of the class of the 'worst cases', the 'low grades', the 'undeserving poor'.

(Brown and Smith 1989: 108)

Nonetheless, the experience of such groups has enabled more diverse cultures to flourish. They signal the end of assimilation as a goal and suggest an assertive way of challenging more powerful groups to acknowledge and tolerate difference.

In the 1990s, the shift in emphasis from 'mainstreaming' to 'self-help' not only marks disillusionment with a failed strategy but a response to changing material circumstances. Dominant cultural norms have not diversified in the last twenty years, as those in the change movements had hoped or anticipated, they have instead retrenched. Wealth has been aggregated among fewer people and social welfarism has been under sustained attack. People in positions of power are less likely now than at any time in the last fifty years to advocate equality as a social goal, or to believe in the redistribution of wealth. It can be argued, therefore, that the real motives behind new social policies have been obscured by the rhetoric of community care. As Rich (1986) argues,

> The working mother with briefcase was, herself, a cosmetic touch on a society deeply resistant to fundamental changes. The 'public' and 'private' spheres were still in disjunction. She had not found herself entering into an evolving new society, a society in transformation. She had only been integrated into the same structures which had made liberation movement necessary. It was not the Women's Liberation Movement that had failed to 'solve anything'. There had been a counter revolution and it had absorbed her.
>
> (Rich 1986: xiv)

Given that the pervasive cultural norms, which value competitiveness, intelligence, individualism and acquisitiveness, are inimical to people with disabilities, there are some groups, notably religious foundations, who promote alternative values which respect people with disabilities and undertake to care for and with them, in defiance of the 'world outside'. Interestingly such communities often run without hierarchies, in rural settings where people with different abilities can contribute to the fabric of community life (Robinson 1989). Such an approach is inconsistent with the normalisation principle but consistent with its goal of providing valued social roles for people with disabilities. As Robinson argues (ibid.: 250) such groups provide segregation with the goal of protecting a higher quality of life for people with disabilities. In a diverse culture, where the dominant values oppress people with disabilities, it seems likely that they might group together to resist and that people who value them should also group together to live a life which includes and respects them. This might, of course, be the meaning of asylum in the next decade – the ability of such groups to protect themselves and their values without walls.

Normalisation, like feminism, is often posited as being neither politically right nor left wing: the difference, however, is fundamental to any movement seeking to re-establish people with disabilities in valued roles in society. Right-wing philosophy rests on a hierarchy which is either based on birth or merit, while left-wing ideologies are based on the notion of equal rights for all, regardless of race, creed or class. The position of people with disabilities in a right-wing society inevitably depends on charity: in a left-wing society, disabled people can assert their rights to be treated equitably with other citizens.

Being in receipt of charity or pity is, ipso facto, accepting a socially devalued role. The spectacle of the television telethons brought disabled people out in protest at the demeaning images and stereotypical presentation of their issues, images which undermine respectful attitudes within the community, even as they purport to raise funds for community care. Ruth Hill, writing in *The Observer*, speculates:

> How many people who donate to the Spastics Society or took part in a sponsored throwing-custard-pies at Nicholas Parsons' session for Telethon, would also virulently oppose a scheme for people with learning difficulties next door to them?
>
> (*The Observer*: 2.9.90)

The new imagery conjured up by such events has replaced the horrors of the institution. The spectacle of members of the public organising trivial games and silly pursuits as an answer to people in pain, poverty or distress disguises the real source of that distress in policies which have taken from these groups a proper share of resources and testifies to the depth of their marginalisation. It encapsulates indignity in a form of light entertainment, a twentieth-century Nero's circus.

The normalisation movement must tackle these new manifestations of the old imagery and analyse the new rhetoric. Constant references to consumerism emerge in recent policy documents and reflect an ideological shift about the transfer of services from the public to the private sector. The assumption that the market place offers the best safeguards for service users is central to the health services reforms of the late 1980s in the United Kingdom (HMSO 1989). Describing service users as consumers evades the immense vulnerability and dependence on services of the people themselves. As Winkler (1987) notes, the analogy of an individual with disabilities as supermarket shopper is false:

The supermarket vision of customer relations extends to reducing the waits at the check out counter and exchanging faulty goods with the minimum of questions asked. It does not extend (even at Marks and Spencers) to inviting the customers on to the board, nor to consulting them about investment or even about what should be on the shelves, let alone in their products. The supermarket concept certainly does not mean that retailers help customers sue manufacturers of products which have caused them harm.

(Winkler 1987)

Clearly people with disabilities do not interact with the community care agencies in the role of discerning shoppers who can take their business elsewhere if they fail to get satisfaction. It is even unclear, as new forms of privatised care develop, whether they are actually being offered the role of consumer with its illusion of power – perhaps their real status is as commodities who can be bought and sold alongside the fixtures and fittings of the homes they inhabit on the owners' terms.

The only way for the goal of 'ordinariness' to be achieved is if people with disabilities share with other ordinary people the right to housing, income maintenance, health, educational and leisure services, and that they are able to secure these rights in an unobtrusive way. That is essentially a radical agenda.

NORMALISATION AND VALUING WOMEN WHO USE SERVICES

If, as we argue above, there are significant conflicts in the normalisation principle when viewed from a feminist point of view, there is a need to examine how these conflicts affect women who use services directly, or as relatives and carers of people with disabilities. Women with learning difficulties and women with mental health problems share a common experience as women whose needs services have been slow to address. But the failure of these women to conform to culturally valued notions also penalises them in different ways and juxtaposing them hides important differences, just as paying insufficient attention to class and ethnicity undermined early feminist thinking about the nature of oppression and led to simplistic, individually based strategies for change.

Women with learning difficulties form a distinct group who are caught by the conflicts inherent in normalisation. New services have tended to imitate the nuclear family in grouping people together in small houses, women in these groups are likely to find themselves in a 'housekeeping' role, in this case servicing men whom they have not chosen and with whom they do not have close personal ties. They are, like other women, vulnerable to domestic or sexual violence in such settings, yet services have rarely attended to issues of protection in a serious way. The need to protect women from abuse may be sacrificed to the more urgent service requirement of keeping open a placement for a difficult male client. Services which have a clearer understanding of vulnerability, in terms of power and oppression would make a more unequivocal commitment to protecting women (and vulnerable men) from harassment or violence.

However, this is a catch 22 situation because although services have reproduced these pseudo-family groups the reality has proved elusive. Services have made little progress towards assisting women with disabilities in taking on the roles of wife and mother. The 'valued' model of a separate couple managing alone is one which heightens individual difficulties and minimises support and may have obstructed services from seeking this option for women with learning difficulties. Equally, lesbian relationships are not valued by the wider society and within normalisation may be seen to disadvantage women with disabilities further. However, such relationships might offer them a chance of equal power and nurturance.

The Scandinavian approach (Perrin and Nirje 1985: 71) which emphasises choice rather than conformity is more consistent with a strategy to open up alternative lifestyles and more assertive routes to empowerment. While Wolfensberger argues that subjective notions such as happiness should not necessarily be the goal for service users (see Lindley and Wainwright, this volume), we would argue that any alternative assumes that one party, be it professional, policy maker or normalisation devotee, can authoritatively claim to know what is best for the other. Any situation in which an individual or group's subjective experience is discounted in favour of an 'objective' account of what they feel, think or want clearly signals an abuse of power.

Some people with disabilities will necessarily need others to be involved in making significant decisions about their lives. Operating on the basis of 'What would this person do if they valued themselves?' as opposed to 'What would this person do if they are to be valued by others?' would go some way towards incorporating a subjective stance, even where the person is unable to speak for themselves. This approach would provide a way of challenging, rather than perpetuating, situations which people have been taught to want by the devaluing experiences they have endured. Thus a person who says they would rather stay in a large, inhumane institution could be moved on the grounds that if they valued themselves, they would not want to live there. Similarly, services would not condone violent or abusive relationships on the grounds that women with disabilities were 'choosing' them. Thus it would fall within the remit of services to support a 'valuing' rather than a 'valued' lifestyle for people where the two are not synonymous.

There are services which have helped women to present themselves more positively, nevertheless women with disabilities will often fall short of the idealised and stereotyped standards of attractiveness laid down for all women. This makes it difficult for individual women to acquire a strong sense of their own bodies. Women with learning difficulties can come up against a silence that makes it difficult for them to learn skills or develop a positive sense of their sexuality. Menstruation will be dealt with as a toileting chore rather than as a significant life event; they may not see 'valued' women managing their periods because to manage successfully in Western cultures means to manage in secret. Masturbation is also an area where misconceptions about what is normal or what is valued will discriminate against women, especially those with learning difficulties. Discussion about teaching individuals to masturbate focuses almost exclusively on men and sexual frustration is attributed to them more readily.

Some services have begun to recognise that women's groups are a valued and valuable option which enable women with disabilities to address these issues for themselves, to ask questions of each other, to talk about their experiences and to challenge the unrealistic norms against which all women are judged. However, 'women only' disability services are not widely available and whereas service users see their care being managed by women, they will usually also see that the real power lies with the (often male) manager. Thus women with disabilities internalise a hierarchy in which they are at a double disadvantage – they see women to whom they aspire, devalued within service organisations. Thus services which, by following normalisation strategies, were hoping to open up options for women with disabilities both failed to challenge the narrow range of roles sanctioned for women, and to provide adequate support for them to take on traditional women's caring or domestic roles within the community. Moreover, they have left women exposed within small group living situations and within the community at large, without adequate protection or precaution against abuse.

Women with mental health problems may face sharper conflicts in a service which is modelling daily living situations on 'valued' and typical models, when these very structures are implicated in the origins of individual women's mental distress. Depression has been shown to be linked to caring for young children in isolated settings (Brown and Harris 1978) while sexual abuse is now known to be implicated in a high proportion of psychiatric referrals (Gil 1988). Furthermore, unacknowledged issues for women, around, for example, miscarriage or abortion, infertility or menopause, tend to be framed in terms of illness or imbalance, when distress is clearly a legitimate response to what are significant losses and life events. Every data source shows more women than men diagnosed as having mental illness (see Howell and Baynes 1981: 155). When women come together around these issues they discover that they are not in fact 'deviant'. What is deviant in Western cultures is the drawing of attention towards women's real issues and experience in an open and explicit way. Self-help groups are now the preferred method of treatment for many women who have experienced abuse or incest (Hall and Lloyd 1989), as well as for women who have been labelled depressed, agoraphobic or who refer themselves for various eating disorders (see Orbach 1978).

Normalisation, in its analysis of institutional experience, added a helpful spur to the resistance of service users and workers to pathologising individuals who are being devalued. But its emphasis on conformity undermines this strategy for women who are caught in a vicious circle, in that their devaluation springs from their experience as women and is then compounded by the label of mental illness which serves to disguise the real oppression they have suffered.

If we adopt the strategy of enabling individual women to value themselves, rather than attempt to accommodate to culturally valued norms, a different agenda would emerge. This would allow women who use services to acknowledge and protect themselves from sexual violence, to receive services in which they are not further disempowered by professional and hierarchical relationships, to make communal living and childcare arrangements at certain periods of their lives and to have the support of other women in addressing health care issues. Such a strategy immediately calls into question prevailing values and service structures.

Thus we can see that women are both disabled by their oppression as women and doubly at a disadvantage because as disabled women they have to live within the confines of two sets of devaluing expectations. Normalisation does not provide a framework for addressing the actual day-to-day experiences of being devalued. At best it makes some material improvements; at worst, it creates an elaborate pretence which blocks individuals from recognising what has happened to them.

VALUING WOMEN WHO ACT AS CARERS

Because the focus of normalisation is the individual experiences of people with disabilities, it has had little to say about the role of carers, although Wolfensberger (1987) explicitly values unpaid help over paid care. As Pascall (1986) points out, married women are the 'only large group whose labour is no charge to public expenditure', so it is to them that such an exhortation must have been addressed. The only other insight within normalisation which has a bearing on the disproportionate share of caring work undertaken by women is the notion of 'deviancy juxtaposition' which predicts that low-status people, such as people with disabilities, will find themselves being cared for by other low-status groups, most notably women and black workers. In a very real sense, people with disabilities find themselves corralled with women in 'female' environments, most usually with women relatives at home. The juxtaposition is neither accidental nor illusory – it is rooted in the economic imperative to keep care in the private rather than the public domain.

A cynical view of the success of the normalisation movement might start by calling its bedfellows into question. While radicals within and beyond the movement were using the ideology to work towards the closure of large inhumane institutions, the government was using community care to limit spending on the elderly and handicapped and to 'disguise policies whose real effects are to burden and isolate individuals' (Pascall 1986: 86). The consensus about what the state should provide has shifted through the 1980s, at the expense of women who act as carers. Before this time, the cost of institutional care was borne completely by the state and admission represented a firm demarcation line across which family members did not stray. Admission divested them of both financial and practical responsibility. Recent policies to restrict admissions to long-stay hospitals are now resisted by many parents and carers, not because they support this form of care, but because they know that the alternative is nothing.

Despite the strong commitment of carers to decent and humane services for their family members and the successful promulgation of community care as an ideology (see Dalley, this volume), carers still seek admission to hospital in the face of public policies which declare this option closed. Foster (1987) reports that the parents in her study who were seeking admission to a declining institution in the United States did so because they had defined their situation as intolerable (see also Pahl and Quine 1984). In practice, of course, most carers actively seek to be involved in both the caring relationship and the work which goes with it but they have no rights whatsoever; what they have is what women have always had, 'the power-less responsibility for human lives' (Rich 1986: 277). Delphy (1984), a French economist, sees, in women's work in the home, more the characteristics of indentured labour than of independent economic relations:

> The new analyses show the family as itself the site of economic exploitation: that of women. Having shown that domestic work and childrearing are, first, exclusively the responsibility of women, and, second, unpaid,

these essays conclude that women have a specific relationship to production which is comparable to serfdom.

(Delphy 1984: 59)

Thus women who work outside the home constitute a class of wage earners
while women who do the same task, but in the domestic sphere, have terms
and conditions reminiscent of servants in bygone households.

Meanwhile, normalisation, which has implicitly supported community
care policies, has sidestepped the issue altogether. Only by keeping blinkers
firmly in place could it be argued that people with disabilities are well
served by individuals who have no choice over their involvement and no
power to access resources as they need them. Only the most disinterested
would fail to notice that the bulk of such individuals are women. The Equal
Opportunities Commission (1980, 1982a, 1982b, 1984) has reported that
women make up the overwhelming majority of carers, in the approximate
ratio of three to one. The EOC study (1982a) also unravels the myth that
care is undertaken by any kind of social network. Indeed, it can be seen that
the more difficult the task of caring for a particular individual, the less
likely it is that friends, neighbours or relatives will step in.

The implications of public policy, which is so evidently relying on carers
to avert the system from collapse, are enormous. Changing family patterns,
increased rates of divorce and the upcoming demographic dip – which has
been heralded as a signal for women to return in larger numbers to paid
work outside the home – all question the availability of women to care for
the increasing population of elderly and frail people. Against this backdrop,
normalisation has boosted the appeal of community care, of which Pascall
remarks:

An ideology which romanticises caring for the elderly and the handicapped seems more improbable than one which romanticises motherhood. However, the idea of 'community care', while less developed than
romanticized notions of motherhood, fulfils a very similar function in
legitimating minimal state activity in the private sphere of the home and
family. It also disguises minimal men's activity.

(Pascall 1986: 85)

In recent years, Wolfensberger (1990) has allied himself strongly with
the anti-abortion movement. Ostensibly this expresses an absolute commitment to the rights of the foetus but it operates to further disempower women
and blame them for the conditions in which they have to carry out their
caring responsibilities. The truth is that women make such decisions in a
less than ideal world, one in which they have the welfare of others to
contend with as well as their own stress. Pahl and Quine's (1984) sample of

mothers with children with learning difficulties scored highly on a range of stress measures. The extent of the caring work they do is difficult to countenance, as is the explicit love and tenderness they express for their children. Nevertheless, nine out of ten of the mothers said that, in retrospect, had they been offered the choice they would have chosen to terminate their pregnancies. These mothers are not the evil agents of 'death-making' (Wolfensberger 1990), they are the ones who get up in the night and do the washing, the ones who try to balance the needs of their children with handicaps against those of their other children and their partners whilst mediating between generations, professionals and neighbours.

Normalisation rightly identifies how devaluing it is for people with disabilities to be cast as a burden. But not using the word has not changed the reality. It is otherwise silent about the role and supports which should be offered to women who care, and silent about whether the framework could be used to reverse their own deprivation and devaluation (see Brown and Basset 1991). It speaks neither of – nor to – women who care. We do not see the needs of carers as a competing agenda, vying with those of people with disabilities for validation and resources. We see them as a significant item on the same agenda because feminist social policy has 'been much concerned with dependency ... and with just how tightly the knot has been tied between the dependency of the caring and the dependency of the cared for' (Pascall 1986: 30).

VALUING WOMEN WHO WORK IN SERVICES

Women who work in services have much in common with those who care at home, in that they have little control over the work they do or the resources they have at their disposal. They also have to deal with the realities of sexual inequality in the workplace. The health service is still hidebound by a division of labour which 'gave cure to male doctors and care to female nurses, but it put doctors in charge' (Pascall 1986: 186). Men prescribe, women nurse. Normalisation has contributed its own dynamics to this process. Its emphasis on age- and culture-appropriate language, while designed to revalue people with disabilities, has been used oppressively to rob women of the language they use to describe the work they do. Phrases, such as 'looking after' or 'minding' someone are accurate and respectful; they describe the intuitive balancing which women do when caring for others while attending to their other chores.

Women staff are thus disadvantaged in their dealings with men in hierarchies; their own experience of 'managing' within the home being explicitly devalued while their experience of 'being managed' in the work setting is often disempowering and dehumanising. Booth (1988) comments on the fact that the commitment to revalue people with disabilities is often voiced by individuals who are vociferously defending their own position within occupational hierarchies, their commitment to righting the gross inequality suffered by people with disabilities remaining insulated from any more global 'principle of equality' (ibid.: 116). Thus, although normalisation is claimed to be universally applicable, it is not used explicitly to ensure that part-time workers are accorded equal status to full-time workers. It has not been used to challenge the poor working conditions of ancillary workers and cleaners on recently privatised cleaning contracts. Women workers have particular cause to be suspicious of the rhetoric of 'valuing' people in services when they are so signally devalued as a group themselves.

Professionalisation has not provided a useful framework for most women, even though it has seemingly liberated a few. This is qualified by the fact that 'women's' professions are downgraded as a whole, as in the case of speech therapists, physiotherapists and nurses. The Griffiths Report (1988) paved the way for the government to assume that inexperienced and unskilled young people, in the form of the new community care workers, will be able to do what is only, after all, women's work. Professionalisation has done little to challenge the assumption that women's work is, of itself, unskilled and unworthy. Wolfensberger's view (1987) that only personal relationships could offer any genuine connection for people with disabilities denies the resilience of individual women to care despite, rather than because of, service structures, and further devalues the status of caring and women's rights to proper recompense. We would agree with Wolfensberger, though, that conditions within which women and men can care coherently for people with disabilities and for each other are rarely found in human services. Professional stature ensures that (for some) the work involved is rightly seen as complex and demanding but professional structures divide and disempower both workers and users.

AN AGENDA FOR FUTURE ACTION

As feminist women who have been influenced by normalisation and who, in turn, want to influence it, we would suggest the following agenda for the movement in the 1990s: an agenda which changes the emphasis but not, we believe, the fundamental humanism inherent in the original principle. The list is in order of priority; it represents a hierarchy, but unlike most hierarchies it starts with those who have the least power.

First, that we actively support, empower, encourage and facilitate what we have called 'meaningful association' between people with disabilities, in and through self-help groups, consciousness-raising groups, user management of services and visible political activity and campaigning by people with disabilities for the resources which they decide are most important to them. This support should take the form of securing funding, time, space (that is, rooms and the right to chosen segregation) and, where asked for, facilitation in the form of group skills. It will require great sensitivity for professionals to help such groups without turning them into puppet planning groups or structures which are dominated by professionals. Nonetheless, skilled help may be needed by groups who have not traditionally had the power to keep others out, to set boundaries around their time, space and the tasks they want to accomplish. Once set the helper needs to withdraw and respect those boundaries, reverting to the role of outsider.

This overturns the imperative in normalisation to value relationships with non-disabled people above those which are forged out of recognising and respecting shared experience and identity. It asserts that one can only value oneself if one is able to value others who are like oneself. It rejects as a route to empowerment the uncomfortable accommodation of being the 'token', the minority who is always the least powerful.

Second, that professionals take seriously the need to protect vulnerable people from abuse within service systems and within the community at large. This is not an optional extra, or an individual trauma which should be suppressed in the interests of some wider or longer term goal (as it always is if women protest against pornography, rape or domestic violence). It is the very essence of what it means to be devalued. Instead of inviting people to hide their experiences of victimisation in the belief that such disavowal will protect the ideals of community care, professionals should ally themselves with individuals who have been abused, insulted or deprived of basic rights and help them to make this knowledge public. This confronts the 'community' and insists that they acknowledge what is done to people with disabilities in their midst.

It also involves protesting about facilities which are not made accessible, boycotting pubs which ask people with disabilities to leave, using the local press and media skilfully and where these impose some form of censorship, going directly to the people who are customers, neighbours and so on, to get their support in the face of apathy or rejection. Sometimes such a campaign will necessitate using the courts to validate the person with a disability and seek redress on their behalf, thus making clear that the commitment to protecting people with disabilities from physical and sexual abuse is unequivocal. The experience of women and children suggests that this can only be attempted (let alone achieved!) in a climate which acknowledges that such abuse exists and that its victims speak the truth.

Third, normalisation is silent about carers but we believe that any movement which aims to enhance the quality of life for people with disabilities and to safeguard their rights should make the deprivation of those who directly do the community's work of caring a legitimate focus for concern and action. We want the reality of caring to be made public and political, to encourage the women who do this work to speak out without feeling guilty or disloyal. We urge professionals who work in the field of community care to unite to create political pressure for real changes in the material circumstances of their lives. A charter of carers' rights should be drawn up which makes clear demands for income maintenance and support and insists that such provision is framed, not only to ensure that women are not discriminated against, but that these benefits actively recognise the fact that it is women who are doing this work and that they will not have had so-called 'typical', uninterrupted working lives. Benefits which are accessed by reference to previous length of employment are not going to help women who give up their jobs to care for relatives any more than they help women who have been effectively barred from entering the workforce in the first place. Credit for pension schemes and so on, are the least that women should be asked to accept for their willingness to do this work. Such a charter should set minimum guidelines for the hours in a week which carers are allowed to work without respite, the number of disturbed nights in each month which they are allowed to endure without support and the free time in each year to which they are entitled for the pursuit of their own health and happiness. If ever there was a case for protective employment legislation it is for the women who care, carry, clean, affirm, bathe, feed, entertain, nurse, teach and keep patience with people with disabilities while attending to the needs of other family members and mediating between generations, siblings, neighbours and professionals.

For the movement to take on board such a commitment implies a shift of focus from the individual with disabilities to the context within which he or she is cared for. We believe that without an analysis which supports the humanity of the carer there is always a pull towards them being blamed or scapegoated. Such respite as is given to carers should be collective and flexible, wherever possible within their control and accessible without the indignity of means tests and professional assessments. Developing structures which can help carers, who have traditionally been isolated from each other, to sustain each other should be seen as an important concomitant of this commitment.

Finally, paid carers are also in need of revaluing – we propose that any movement for people with disabilities should vigorously pursue improved conditions and remuneration without being compromised by vague notions of personal sacrifice or confused by critiques of professionalisation. The current hourly rate for the jobs which involve caring directly for people, as opposed to managing or co-ordinating services, is so low that it will be a long time before we have to worry about the prospect of people entering the field for greed. The gulf between these so-called 'basic grade' workers, who are overwhelmingly women and 'professionally qualified' staff, who are sometimes women, should be lessened by valuing the former upwards. This will require an accurate description of the demands of the work and the skill needed to do it, the utmost care in the language used to describe the people who do the caring work and a consistent refusal to scapegoat or blame them. The inclusion of real caring work in the job descriptions of the highly paid, whether they be professionals, managers, entrepreneurs or academics, should be encouraged.

The normalisation movement should draw on its understanding to attend to the way such jobs are reframed and revalued. Again we favour the use of collective routes to re-establish the worthiness of caring jobs, through trade unions, contract specification relating to equal opportunities and minimum wage rates, broader access to training and development opportunities and very visible complaints and negotiation procedures.

This agenda differs in emphasis from that set out by Wolfensberger in the 1970s and 1980s in two important ways. First, it is concerned to recognise both cared for and carers as victims of the community's lack of coherent commitment to the lives of people with disabilities. Second, it is an agenda which asserts the importance of communal and collective solutions, because these challenge rather than collude with prevailing values, values which essentially work against people with disabilities and their families. We cannot continue to ask people uncritically to conform to the very values which are responsible for their being on the scrapheap in the first place. Thus we favour public rather than private change and communal rather than privatised structures.

We wish that we could have drawn up this agenda in a spirit of optimism but the 1990s are not beginning in that vein. Recession is promised and in recession, women and people with disabilities suffer first. The mixed economy of care may prove exploitative of users, carers and workers as the slender protection offered by national agreements and policy guidelines are dismantled and the new mechanisms of contracting and local employment negotiations are introduced. We wish that, as non-disabled feminists, we could have said to people with disabilities, their carers and those who work with them 'Look, we have found that this really works as an effective strategy . . do this and you will find yourself taken notice of, valued, in charge of your lives . . .', but we cannot say that. We have to draw the conclusion that working together will probably not have much impact given the priorities and ideology of those in power but we see it as the only way to fight back from a position of self-respect. We would probably have to say something along the lines of 'Forget culturally valued norms! You are not valued in this society and by this economy – resist visibly, but most of all resist together!'.

REFERENCES

Atkinson, D., and Ward, L. (1987) 'A part of the community: Social integration and neighbourhood networks', *Talking Points* 3, London: CMH.

Booth, T. (1988) 'Challenging conceptions of integration', in L. Barton (ed.) *The Politics of Special Educational Needs*, Lewes: Falmer Press.

Brown, G., and Harris, T. (1978) *The Social Origins of Depression*, London: Tavistock.

Brown, H. (1983) 'Why is it such a big secret? Sex education for handicapped young adults', in A. Craft and M. Craft (eds) *Sex Education and Counselling for Mentally Handicapped People*, Tunbridge Wells: Costello.

Brown, H., and Bassett, T. (1991) *New Lifestyles for Carers: A training exercise based on the normalisation principle*, Brighton: Pavilion Publishing.

Brown, H., and Smith, H. (1989) 'Whose "ordinary" life is it anyway? – a feminist critique of the normalisation principle', *Disability, Handicap and Society* 4, 2: 105–19.

Dalley, G. (1988) *Ideologies of Caring – rethinking community and collectivism*, London: MacMillan Education.

Delphy, C. (1984) *Close to Home – a materialist analysis of women's oppression*, London: Hutchinson.

Dworkin, A. (1981) *Pornography – men possessing women*, London: Women's Press.

Dworkin, A. (1986) *Letters from a War Zone*, London: Secker and Warburg.

Edgar, D. (1987) 'The morals dilemma', *Marxism Today* October.

Equal Opportunities Commission (1980) *The Experience of Caring for Elderly and Handicapped Dependants: A survey report*.

Equal Opportunities Commission (1982a) *Caring for the Elderly and Handicapped: Community care and women's lives*.

Equal Opportunities Commission (1982b) *Who Cares for the carers? Opportunities for those caring for the elderly and handicapped*.

Equal Opportunities Commission (1984) *Carers and Services: A comparison of men and women caring for dependent elderly people*.

Flynn, M. (1987) 'Independent living arrangements for adults who are mentally handicapped', in N. Malin (ed.) *Reassessing Community Care*, London: Routledge.

Foster, S. (1987) *The Politics of Caring*, Lewes: Falmer Press.

Friedan, B. (1963) *The Feminine Mystique*, Harmondsworth: Penguin.

Gil, E. (1988) *Treatment of Adult Survivors of Child Abuse*, Walnut Creek: Launch Press.

Goffman, E. (1961) *Asylum*, Harmondsworth: Penguin.

Griffiths Report (1988) *Community Care: An Agenda for Action*, London: HMSO.

Hall, L., and Lloyd, S. (1989) *Surviving Child Sexual Abuse*, Lewes: Falmer Press.

Hill, R. (1990) 'Grant us some dignity before your donations', *Observer* 2 September: 55.

HMSO (1989) *Caring for People: Community care in the next decade and beyond*, CM849.

Howell, E., and Baynes, M. (1981) *Women and Mental Health*, New York: Basic Books.

O'Brien, J. (1987) 'A guide to lifestyle planning', in B. Wilcox and G. Bellamy (eds) *The Activities Catalogue: An alternative curriculum for youth and adults with severe disabilities*, Baltimore: Brooke.

Oliver, M. (1988) 'The social and political context of educational policy', in L. Barton (ed.) *The Politics of Special Educational Needs*, Lewes: Falmer Press.

Orbach, S. (1978) *Fat is a Feminist Issue*, New York: Berkely Publishing.

Pahl, J., and Quine, L. (1984) *Families with Mentally Handicapped Children: A study of stress and of service response*, University of Kent at Canterbury: Health Services Research Unit.

Pascall, G. (1986) *Social Policy: A feminist analysis*, London: Tavistock.

Perrin, B., and Nirje, B. (1985) 'Setting the record straight: A critique of some frequent misconceptions of the normalisation principle', *Australian and New Zealand Journal of Developmental Disabilities* 11: 69–74.

Rich, A. (1986) *Of Woman Born – motherhood as experience and institution*, New York: W.W. Norton.

Robinson, T. (1989), 'Normalisation: The whole answer?', in A. Brechin and J. Walmsley (eds) *Making Connections*, Milton Keynes: Open University Press.

Sinason, V. (1986) 'Secondary mental handicap and its relationship to trauma', *Psychoanalytic Psychotherapy* 2, 2: 131–54.

Szivos, S., and Griffiths, E. (1990) 'Consciousness raising and social identity theory: A challenge to normalisation', *Forum* 28, August: 11–15.

Tajfel, H. (1981) *Human Groups and Social Categories*, Cambridge: Cambridge University Press.

Walmsley, S. (1989) 'The need for safeguards', in H. Brown and A. Craft (eds) *Thinking the Unthinkable – papers on sexual abuse and people with learning difficulties*, London: FPA.

Weeks, J. (1989) 'Aids, altruism and the New Right', in E. Carter and S. Watney (eds) *Taking Liberties – Aids and cultural politics*, London: Serpent's Tail.

Winkler, F. (1987) 'Consumerism in health care: Beyond the supermarket model', *Policy and Politics* 15, 7.

Wolfensberger, W. (1987) 'How to Function with Personal Moral Coherency in a Disfunctional (Human Service) World', Workshop offered by the Training Institute for Human Service Planning and Change Agentry, Syracuse University, New York.

Wolfensberger, W. (1990) 'A most critical issue: Life or death', *Changes* March, 8: 1.

Wolfensberger, W., and Tullman, S. (1989) 'A brief outline of the principle of normalisation', in A. Brechin and J. Walmsley (eds) *Making Connections*, Milton Keynes: Open University.

Postscript

Hilary Brown and Helen Smith

Readers may be divided about the capacity for and/or the desirability of normalisation remaining as a leading model for community care into the 1990s: uncertain if the initial impetus it created can be maintained or whether the contradictions and inconsistencies described in this book indicate that the theory has 'had its day'. Certainly the criticisms levelled at normalisation by various authors, both here and elsewhere, have to be faced rather than bounced back, incorporated rather than deflected.

To do this, a more diffuse network will need to be fostered and one within which ownership of the ideas is not so tightly defined. The manner in which the theory has been disseminated has been as contentious as the ideas themselves. Much of the debate and critique has focused on one man and his undeniable influence over a theory that has shaped services for people with disabilities in countries such as the United States, Canada, Britain, Australia and New Zealand. The early origins of normalisation in Scandinavia and Denmark are often forgotten or obscured by the stamp of Wolfensberger's personality and ideas which have become the trademark of contemporary formulations of normalisation in this country.

The traditions and structures of power, which have enabled such a strong identification between Wolfensberger, the man, and normalisation, the theory, to emerge, are in themselves problematic. His supporters have stressed the need to maintain control over a set of ideas, the challenging nature of which made them open to attack and distortion. His detractors have seen this control as yet another form of the very oppression normalisation seeks to overcome. In a more democratic debate, we must all take responsibility for the way in which we interpret and use the ideas to develop more appropriate and valuing services for people with disabilities. Recourse to an 'expert' is not a substitute for the moral responsibility which we all have, responsibility proportionate to the power we can exercise in bringing about change.

Meanwhile, people with disabilities are immensely vulnerable to the whims and dictates of an uncaring and intolerant society. Their power-lessness has resulted in them being segregated and discriminated against, warehoused in intolerable conditions, kept in poverty in the community or even killed (as in Nazi Germany). Wolfensberger identifies a societal trend towards deathmaking that is targeted primarily at those whose 'deviancy', in the form of physical or mental impairment, marks them out as 'different' (Wolfensberger 1990). He argues persuasively that without the personal commitment of non-disabled citizens, people with disabilities are increas-ingly at risk.

Yet normalisation, in its directive to pursue a valued lifestyle, seems to others to maintain the powerlessness of people with disabilities by restrict-ing individual choice to that which is culturally prescribed as 'valued' and to commend this to people with disabilities as the only way to bring about a change in their status. Mao Tse-tung (1965), in describing how to liberate an oppressed people, states that there are two essential principles under-pinning change:

> one is the actual needs of the masses rather than what we fancy they need, and the other is the wishes of the masses, who must make up their own minds instead of our making up their minds for them.
>
> (Mao Tse-tung 1965: 235)

If normalisation is to take the oppression of people with disabilities into the political arena, it must untangle these different strands, challenging pro-fessional and cultural values which stand in the way. To obscure, rather than to clarify, the conflicts of interest at the heart of services to people with disabilities puts at risk their real liberation.

It seems likely that controversy will continue. Wolfensberger's recent alignment with the anti-abortion lobby and the strength of his view of the world as a place which actively seeks to destroy those labelled as disabled (Wolfensberger 1990) provoke strong reactions. The logical extension of his beliefs that statutory services are intrinsically damaging understandably finds many followers among those who have used or had contact with services but does not provide a strategy, nor the required optimism, to move us towards humane and empowering services.

Many would now agree with the dictate of normalisation that we should be moving away from an 'individual pathology' model towards a paradigm in which disability is perceived as a cultural entity that exists within a specified set of social conditions. Rubin *et al.* (quoted in Oliver 1990), in a study of the Navajo Indians, found a high incidence of limping caused by congenital hip disease. However, as the Indians did not perceive this to be a disability and there was no associated stigma or discrimination, they refused modern medical treatment. Whereas most people with disabilities would heartily commend such an example as evidence of the social construction of disability, in Western capitalist societies in particular, stigma, prejudice and real disadvantage cannot be overcome by simply abolishing services and hoping that by not acknowledging disability, oppression will disappear.

The essence of normalisation – enabling people with disabilities to attain that which most non-disabled people expect as of right – can be seen to be a product of its time, mirroring other social movements of the 1970s. These also advocated a kind of equality based on emulating powerful and advantaged groups (see Whitehead, this volume). In this sense, many of the contributors in this book are arguing for a parallel development of normalisation, commensurate with the development of other social movements (such as the Women's or Black movement) which encourage self-determination and overt resistance to circumscribed and limiting roles. This would necessitate a radical review of the process of 'co-opting' people into valued roles in favour of their positively redefining a role in society which explicitly acknowledges the nature of their 'difference', reversing Wolfensberger's belief that

> for the largest number of devalued persons, the *right not to be different* in certain dimensions of living is actually a much more urgent issue than the right to be different.
>
> (Wolfensberger 1980: 93, original emphasis)

Thus, new formulations of normalisation must be enhanced by a consideration of gender and ethnicity (see Ferns, this volume).

There are also ways in which normalisation can be furthered by technical improvements in our skills (for example, developing links with behavioural therapy, as discussed by McGill and Emerson, this volume). This would require that the normalisation movement suspend its ideological purity and realise that a values-base can usefully inform other techniques rather than be compromised by them. It also requires such technologies to recognise the importance of basing any intervention with people with disabilities in principles which respect peoples' worth and abilities. Equally, the practical effects of normalisation, such as 'mainstreaming' and community integration, can be informed and strengthened by a debate with other relevant social psychological theories (see Szivos, this volume) which may usefully challenge some of its assumptions.

The outcomes of normalisation in many services, especially those for people with learning difficulties, have been great. It has had an important role in sensitising service providers and others in society to the injustices in the lives of people with disabilities and has proved a powerful tool for raising consciousness amongst professionals. On the other hand, it could be argued that a key to its popularity is that it offers guidelines for action about inequality which do not call into question their own positions of power. The alleged inadequacy of normalisation theorists seriously to acknowledge the centrality of power and powerlessness in the lives of those who provide and use human services is common to many other theories that inform the work of people in the caring professions (Williams and Watson 1991a).

Proponents of normalisation may challenge whether the issue of power, one that has been raised in many different ways in this book, is a legitimate focus of study, and may assert that empowerment will naturally follow if the principles are adhered to. Critics, though, will claim that people working in the caring professions need theories that explicitly sensitise them to the social and social psychological processes which create and maintain social inequalities – relying on 'common sense' to guide work on empowerment is a risky business in a culture which is structured by social inequalities based on class, gender and race. As Baker-Miller and Mothner note,

> our lives are so affected by irrational inequalities, we are so busy denying and falsifying them, that we do not know how to deal with those who are truly not equal in certain respects.
>
> (Baker-Miller and Mothner 1981: 84)

The implications for service users of this limitation in normalisation have been well documented here. The implications for professionals is that they may get job satisfaction from apparently working in the best interests of clients, while their own position and power largely remain unexamined and unaffected. Workers in human services need concepts or models to help them grapple with the *dynamics* of change, both within their own relationships with service users, carers and less valued staff and in the context of attempted social integration.

So what needs to change? First, we need to recognise the strengths of normalisation, that is, its focus on the oppression in the lives of people with disabilities and the importance attached to their gaining equality in terms of access to 'rights' and resources. We need to rethink the importance attached to 'roles' and 'value' against the backdrop of our patriarchal culture and question whether these work in the interests of service users, acknowledging explicitly where there *is* a conflict of interests. We need to learn how to empower consumers to make decisions about the values and rules that control their personal and collective future by listening to them directly but also by drawing widely from a wide range of relevant literatures, for example, novels, autobiographies, feminist theories and research (see

Brown and Smith, this volume; Williams and Watson 1991b), work in social psychology (Apfelbaum 1978), social policy (see Dalley, this volume) and elsewhere throughout the humanities and social sciences. Moreover, if normalisation is to move beyond its current parameters and seriously address issues of oppression and injustice, it must inevitably have an impact on the lives of professionals, raising fundamental questions about their knowledge base and identities. It should inform decisions about remuneration, for both formal and informal carers, challenging traditional career paths for different grades and types of workers.

As a social movement normalisation *has* achieved success in terms of putting the issue of 'disabling' services on the agenda of many health, local authority and voluntary organisations, and this, of itself, may ensure that it has a continuing role to play in the 1990s. Some contributors (such as Tyne, and McGill and Emerson, this volume) have pointed out the way normalisation has sometimes been used to lend credence to bad practice, to justify a non-interventionist approach where helping the individual is testing our capacities to the limit. New services must gain confidence in learning from their mistakes and, rather than referring back to received wisdom, create ways of clarifying what is actually happening in the lives of service users and how change can be achieved. We have to deal with issues of quality by refining our ability to measure and document service outcomes (both quantitatively and qualitatively) so that we are not thrown back on justifying poor services or producing impressionistic judgements, which hide the fact that we are following the letter, but not the spirit of normalisation.

What does normalisation now have to do in order to be a positive force for change in the 1990s? The answer may lie in going back to its roots and realigning itself in relation to other sociological theories. Finklestein (quoted in Oliver 1990) has defined three evolutionary phases in the paradoxical relationship between the state of the individual with a disability (that is, his or her impairment) and the state of society:

> Phase 1 in which disabled individuals formed part of a larger underclass. Phase 2 which saw them separated from their class origins to become a special, segregated group, leading to the paradox whereby disability came to be regarded both as an individual impairment and a social restriction. Phase 3, which is just beginning, sees the end of the paradox whereby disability comes to be perceived solely as social restriction.
>
> (Oliver 1990: 28)

The paradox referred to by Finklestein defines the interaction between a person with disabilities and society in terms which reflect the relationship between individual workers and the economic mode of production and is optimistic that new technology will prove a liberating force, particularly for people with physical disabilities. But there is another, collective, sense in which phase three may be emerging. Groups such as Survivors Speak Out (a network of psychiatric system survivors), People First (a self-advocacy group for people with learning difficulties) and the British Council of Organisations of Disabled People in Britain and their equivalents in the United States and other countries have been steadfastly asserting their rights to determine service developments and priorities and challenging their proscribed status in society. Redefining disability as a configuration of limitations 'out there' rather than as personal deficit opens the way for more assertive renegotiation of roles, resources and recognition.

If normalisation is to survive into the 1990s, it is essential that the movement embraces this issue of empowerment, deriving good service practices from the experiences of user groups and learning from them how best to work in ways which do not take over and disable them further. Normalisation has much to offer with its rigorous analysis of how services systematically devalue individuals and much to learn from people with disabilities, about what it would take to support them in living a life of their own choice.

We would like to thank Dr Jennie Williams, University of Kent, for her help in writing the postscript.

REFERENCES

Apfelbaum, E. (1978) 'Relations of domination and movements for liberation: An analysis of power between groups', in W.G. Austin and S. Worchel (eds) *The Social Psychology of Intergroup Relations*, Montery, California: Brooke/Cole.

Baker-Miller, J., and Mothner, I. (1981) 'Psychological consequences of sexual inequality', in E. Howell and M. Bayes (eds) *Women and Mental Health*, New York: Basic Books.

Mao Tse-tung (1965) *The Selected Works of Mao Tse-tung*, 3, 'The united front in cultured work', Peking: Foreign Language Press.

Oliver, M. (1990) *The Politics of Disablement*, London: Macmillan.

Williams, J., and Watson, G. (1991a) 'Sexual inequality and Clinical Psychology training: Survey report', *Feminism and Psychology* 1, 1.

Williams, J., and Watson, G. (1991b) 'Sexual inequality and Clinical Psychology training: Workshop report', *Feminism and Psychology* 1, 1.

Wolfensberger, W. (1980) 'The definition of normalization – update, problems, disagreements, and misunderstandings', in R. Flynn and K. Nitsch (eds) *Normalization, Integration, and Community Services*, Austin, Texas: Pro-ed.

Wolfensberger, W. (1990) 'A most critical issue: Life or death?', *Changes* 8, 1: 63–73.

Name index

Aanes, D. 63
Abberley, P. 89
Abel, T.M. 117
Abraham, C. 117
Alcoe, J. 28
Allderidge, P. 88
Allen, D. 13
Allen, P. 119
Altmeyer, B.K. 68
Anninson, J.E. 1
Apfelbaum, E. 176
Archer, J. 117, 118
Armstrong, P.M. 62
Atkinson, D. 153
Ayllon, T. 61
Azrin, N.H. 61, 62

Baer, D.M. 61, 66, 67, 68
Bailey, J.S. 62
Baker, M. 66
Baker-Miller, J. 175
Baldwin, S. 20, 63, 75, 77
Balla, D.A. 117
Bank-Mikkelson, N. xvii, 1–3, 6, 110
Banton, M. 135
Baroff, G.S. 117
Bassett, T. 165
Bayley, M.J. 54
Baynes, M. 162
Bean, P. 109
Becker, H. 50
Bellamy, G.T. 61, 62
Benson, B. 121, 124
Bercovici, S.M. 65, 117, 123
Beveridge, W.H. 52
Birenbaum, A. 125

Blakely, E. 69
Blunden, R. 13
Bogdan, R. 8
Bolton, P. 146
Booth, A. xvi
Booth, T. 151, 165, 166
Bourland, G. 68
Braddock, D. 119
Braisby, D. 27, 93, 97
Brickey, M. 125
Briton, J. 115, 121
Brost, M. 71, 92
Brown, G. 97, 161
Brown, H. i, vii, 43, 69, 105, 128; on
    feminist perspective xviii, xxi, 119,
    127, 149–71; on normalisation
    generally xiv–xxii, 172–7; on
    psychodynamic approach xx,
    84–99; on training 27, 28
Brown, P. 4
Bruce, M. 51, 52
Burke, A. 142
Burkhard, J.S. 125
Burleigh, M. 31
Burns, J. 128
Burton, M. 11, 12, 64
Butcher, B.D. 68

Callahan, M. 62, 70, 77
Carr, E.G. 68, 70, 78
Castellani, P.J. 4
Cavalier, A.R. 1
Cheetham, J. 140
Cheseldine, S.E. 125
Clarke, J. 52
Clarke, M. 117, 118, 123

Subject index